The Complete Peanut Allergy Handbook

The Complete
Peanut
Allergy

Handbook

**Everything You Need to Know
to Protect Yourself and Your Child from
the Most Deadly Food Allergy**

Scott H. Sicherer, M.D.,
and Terry Malloy

BERKLEY BOOKS, NEW YORK

THE BERKLEY PUBLISHING GROUP
Published by the Penguin Group
Penguin Group (USA) Inc.
375 Hudson Street, New York, New York 10014, USA

Penguin Group (Canada), 90 Eglinton Avenue East, Suite 700, Toronto, Ontario M4P 2Y3, Canada
(a division of Pearson Penguin Canada Inc.)
Penguin Books Ltd., 80 Strand, London WC2R 0RL, England
Penguin Group Ireland, 25 St. Stephen's Green, Dublin 2, Ireland (a division of Penguin Books Ltd.)
Penguin Group (Australia), 250 Camberwell Road, Camberwell, Victoria 3124, Australia
(a division of Pearson Australia Group Pty. Ltd.)
Penguin Books India Pvt. Ltd., 11 Community Centre, Panchsheel Park, New Delhi—110 017, India
Penguin Group (NZ), Cnr. Airborne and Rosedale Roads, Albany, Auckland 1310, New Zealand
(a division of Pearson New Zealand Ltd.)
Penguin Books (South Africa) (Pty.) Ltd., 24 Sturdee Avenue, Rosebank, Johannesburg 2196,
South Africa

Penguin Books Ltd., Registered Offices: 80 Strand, London WC2R 0RL, England

THE COMPLETE PEANUT ALLERGY HANDBOOK

A Berkley Book / published by arrangement with the author

PRINTING HISTORY
Berkley mass-market edition / August 2005

Copyright © 2005 by Terry Malloy
Cover design by Lesley Worrell
Book design by Kristin del Rosario

The Food Allergy Plan, School Guidelines for Managing Students with Food Allergies, and *How to Read
a Label for a Peanut-Free Diet* are reprinted with permission from FAAN © 2005, The Food Allergy &
Anaphylaxis Network, www.foodallergy.org.

ISBN: 0-425-20441-3

BERKLEY®
Berkley Books are published by The Berkley Publishing Group,
a division of Penguin Group (USA) Inc.,
375 Hudson Street, New York, New York 10014.
BERKLEY is a registered trademark of Penguin Group (USA) Inc.
The "B" design is a trademark belonging to Penguin Group (USA) Inc.

PRINTED IN THE UNITED STATES OF AMERICA

10 9 8 7 6 5 4 3 2 1

To my mentor, Hugh A. Sampson, M.D., and my many medical colleagues and mentors for their wonderful influences. To Anne Muñoz-Furlong, founder of The Food Allergy & Anaphylaxis Network, and all of the individuals who play a role in that organization, having helped more people with food allergy in more ways than can be counted. To all the wonderful people in the Food Allergy Initiative, who are raising money and awareness to improve lives and to cure food allergy. To Sally Noone, R.N., and Shideh Mofidi, M.S., R.D., of the Jaffe Food Allergy Institute for their constant support. To the Jaffe family for having the foresight to establish the Institute. To families living with multiple food allergies and with allergies to foods other than peanut, for forgiving me as I emphasize primarily peanut allergy in this book. (I have not forgotten you, there is a lot in here for you, and I appreciate the unique and difficult challenges that you face.) To my patients from whom I have learned so much and for whom I wish I could do more. And finally, to my wife, Mati, and children, Andrew, Zachary, Maya, Sydnee, and Cassaddee . . . for everything.

—Scott H. Sicherer, M.D.

To Dr. Raghu and Therèse Misra, whose love for each other and for the children in their lives has radiated out and enriched the world.

—Terry Malloy

Contents

Foreword
By Anne Muñoz-Furlong

Dr. Scott Sicherer, in many ways and for many years, has positively affected the lives of thousands of individuals with food allergies. He has spent years researching food allergies, educating the general public and the medical community on the serious nature of food allergies, as well as advocating on behalf of millions of Americans with food allergies for more research and government support of this life-threatening condition.

Families from all parts of the country make the trip to the Mount Sinai School of Medicine in New York City to see him. It is well worth the trip. He listens intently to his patients and combines his medical skills with their information to determine the cause of their illness. He is the perfect person to write this book about an allergy that affects so many and causes fear and stress in daily living for millions of American families.

Dr. Sicherer has taken the hundreds of questions he's heard from patients and their families and condensed them into this book. Whether you want to learn about diagnostic tests, managing peanut allergy in schools, dining out, reaction readiness, or cutting-edge research, it's all here. Wondering how often a severe reaction to peanut is fatal? Or how to find the right doctor? The answers to these questions and more are in this book, too.

Anyone who wants to know more about peanut allergy, including school administrators, child care providers, and family and friends of those with peanut allergy, will find this book a great reference tool that they will go back to over and over again.

Until there is a cure, education is the key to preventing reactions and saving lives. Dr. Sicherer is to be commended for the work he's done on this book to protect patients who have peanut allergy.

Anne Muñoz-Furlong is the Founder and CEO of The Food Allergy & Anaphylaxis Network (FAAN.)

Introduction

After more than a decade of treating children with food allergies, I am frustrated by my inability to provide what can be lifesaving information to everyone who needs it. I know of too many stories where peanut-allergic individuals suffered severe reactions and even fatalities simply because some crucial bit of information was not known or some important advice was not properly followed.

At the same time, my peanut-allergic patients and their families have been consistently educating me and asking me questions, many of them great questions. I have been answering their questions based upon the available medical literature. And when there was no answer in the literature, I have tried to find answers by conducting research studies.

Most of the questions I am asked come from the need to understand peanut allergy and to master living with it until there is a cure. The questions address the many fears and anxieties about living with peanut allergy, how people can successfully cope with this problem, and how they can find a way to enjoy a safe and happy life.

Toward the end of an office visit, I always ask my patients if they have any questions. While many of them have a list, many others, possibly feeling overwhelmed by the problems and complexities of peanut allergy, can't seem to think of any questions. So for them, I both ask the questions and then try to provide the answers. But it never seems enough. So I have often asked myself what else I could do in order to better educate people and help my patients and their families feel more confident and relaxed about dealing with peanut allergy. One of the answers has been writing this book.

With *The Complete Peanut Allergy Handbook*, I hope readers will find that peanut allergy really is manageable. Education is a powerful tool, and until there is a cure for peanut and other food allergies, education will remain the key to success in dealing with this increasingly common allergic disorder.

If you have ordered or purchased this book or if you are in a bookstore trying to decide if it's what you're looking for, please know that every effort was made to be as comprehensive as possible in covering all the questions people ask, or should ask, regarding peanut allergy. This book can be helpful for many people, including:

• Parents of peanut-allergic children;

• Peanut-allergic adults and older children;

• Those who have a family history of peanut and other food allergies;

• Family and friends of peanut-allergic people;

• Current or future school personnel and health care professionals, including teachers, principals, aides, nurses, school bus drivers, emergency medical workers, doctors, paramedics, and any other educational or health care professionals who may work with peanut-allergic children and adults now or in the future;

• Food service workers employed in restaurants, fast-food stores, bakeries, ice cream shops, or anywhere food is provided to the public;

• People who work for companies that manufacture food products, especially those that use peanuts and other nuts in their products; and

• All those who want to be well-informed about a rapidly growing worldwide health concern.

Because peanut allergies are so prevalent today and because they can potentially be life-threatening, we hope this book will provide you with vital information that will help peanut-allergic individuals and all those who know them to feel greater confidence in handling their allergies.

In fact, an estimated 1.7 million Americans suffer from peanut allergies, and day by day, these numbers are growing. For those who are not allergic, peanuts are an everyday part of life, not only as peanut snacks and peanut butter, but as an ingredient in thousands of different foods. An estimated 2.4 billion pounds of peanuts are consumed in the United States every year, with about half in the form of peanut butter. If you're not allergic, peanuts can be a nutritious, enjoyable, and safe part of your diet.

But if you, your child, a relative, or friend has a peanut allergy, for them, even the smallest amount can be life-threatening. Day-to-day living for someone with a peanut allergy is not like that of someone who has no food allergies. People who are sensitive to peanuts have to maintain a lifelong vigilance, making sure to avoid eating peanuts, no matter what the situation. Naturally, this can be stressful, particularly for young peanut-allergic children and their parents.

At first glance, having a peanut allergy sounds pretty upsetting. But as you will see when you read this book, a peanut allergy does not have to ruin anyone's life! People with even the most severe allergies can do everything everyone else does—go to school, play sports, eat in restaurants, attend birthday parties, camp, picnics, and travel—as long as they are well-informed about how to avoid the substance that can cause them serious health problems and always remember to take the proper steps if they are exposed to peanut.

In other words, sometimes it's not the peanut allergy itself that is the biggest danger, it's ignorance of the facts *about* peanut allergy.

We hope that this book will be a handy reference guide for parents of peanut-allergic children, people who have peanut allergies, and all those who know and love them.

This book will tell you:

- What causes an allergy to peanuts

- How you can recognize a peanut allergy

- How to find the right doctor

- What medications are effective and how to use them

- What steps to take when you have an allergic reaction

- How to prevent exposure to peanuts

- Whether tree nuts, such as walnuts or cashews, can also be a problem

- How to shop for safe foods and read labels properly

- What schools, relatives, and friends need to know

- How to select safe restaurants and safe food from their menus

- How to plan a safe vacation

- What to do when you fly with a commercial airline

- Whether peanut allergies are ever outgrown

- What psychological problems can develop and how to deal with them

- How you may prevent peanut allergy

- How to live a happy, normal life when you have a peanut allergy

If you are frequently worried or fearful about your or your child's peanut allergy, you will feel much better when you finish this book. We have tried to cover all the issues that patients have asked about over the years and make it easy for you to understand how peanut allergies develop and what needs to be done so that those who are allergic can remain happy, healthy, and safe.

PLEASE NOTE: In some cases, information has been repeated not only because it relates to more than one chapter but also because we want to reinforce it through repetition. In addition, since every reader has different needs, you may want to skip around the book in order to find the information that is of specific interest to you. We hope this book will become a handy reference for you and your family and friends, providing information whenever you need or want it.

An Introduction to Peanut Allergy

In Part One, you will find out exactly what a peanut allergy is, what causes it, why some people have it and others don't, who is at risk, at what age it may develop, what the common symptoms are, what may be related allergies, and whether or not peanut allergy can be prevented. Most peanut-allergic people want to understand exactly what is going on in their bodies that causes them to react to peanuts, when their friends and other family members have no problem eating peanuts. After reading this section, you will have a very clear idea of what is happening and why.

What Is a Peanut Allergy?

Q: Can we begin by defining what an allergy is?
A: Most of us are familiar with the many common ways in which people experience an "allergic reaction" or an "allergy" to something. There are people who sneeze around cats or during the pollen season, get rashes from certain medications, or, in the case of a food allergy, they may experience symptoms such as rashes or trouble breathing after eating a particular food. In other words, the body has an adverse reaction to something in the environment, such as a food, drug, or other substance to which we are exposed. What really defines an "allergy" is that the immune system, the part of the body designed to fight off infections, is the cause of the problem.

Q: Can you define a peanut allergy?
A: In the case of a peanut allergy, a part of the immune system has recognized the proteins in peanut in a way that results in harmful responses. It is essentially as if the im-

mune system has created an "attack" on the protein. That misdirected attack can harm us in the process.

Q: What happens when the body attacks peanut protein?
A: When the immune system attacks the peanut protein, it produces a substance called an "IgE antibody." An IgE antibody is like a tiny antenna that is able to detect peanut protein. These IgE antibodies sit on the surface of allergy cells that are found in various parts of the body. When you ingest peanut, they capture the peanut protein and alert the allergy cells to release potent chemicals that cause the symptoms of a peanut-allergic reaction.

Q: Why does the body make these IgE antibodies?
A: We do not completely understand why our bodies make these proteins. The parts of the immune system that use these IgE antibodies are the same parts of the immune system that fight parasitic infections, like worms. So it's almost as if the body is ready to attack the types of germs we might encounter in a less westernized or industrialized society, but instead it has directed the attack to harmless peanut proteins. When these IgE antibodies are directed toward airborne proteins like those in pollens, they are responsible for *allergic* diseases, such as hay fever and allergic asthma.

Q: Why do we even have cells that make chemicals causing this allergic reaction?
A: The main cell that packs the chemicals that cause these allergic problems is called a mast cell. This cell captures

and shows the IgE antibody "antenna." We believe that this part of the immune system would normally be ready to kill parasites and may have other functions, but we consider the allergic reaction to foods or to other harmless substances to be a misdirected and overactive response.

Q: Can a person become ill from peanut without being allergic to it?
A: An allergy to food, whether to peanut or other foods, is the result of an immune response to the protein in the food, not to sugars or fats that are also in our food. There are many ways, other than allergy, that we may become sick from a food. For example, if a food spoils we may become ill from toxins released from bacteria. Another example is "intolerance" when there may be a digestive problem for some people associated with the sugars or fats in a food. The best example of intolerance is "lactose intolerance," which happens when a person cannot digest the sugar, called lactose, in milk and milk products, resulting in loose stools. In regard to peanut, this is a fatty food, and some people may not tolerate it well for that reason. Others may have distaste for the flavor or texture. These are not allergies. The major issue in true peanut allergy is that the immune system can be responsible for life-threatening allergic responses to this common food.

Some Important Facts About Peanut Allergy

Q: Approximately how many people have peanut allergy?
A: Based on the studies we performed, in the United States approximately 6 out of 1,000 people in the general population have a peanut allergy. The allergy is more common in children, and approximately 1 out of 125 children has a peanut allergy.

Q: And about how many of these people have what could be termed a "severe" allergy?
A: That is a very tricky question, and the numbers vary by studies done in different countries and how one defines "severe." From our studies, approximately 80 percent of individuals who have a peanut allergy have experienced either a breathing problem associated with a reaction or have experienced problems with multiple areas of their bodies at the same time during a reaction. So this would essentially indicate that about eight out of ten peanut-allergic people have a "severe" peanut allergy.

Q: If you have had a serious problem of this type only once, would you be defined as having a "severe" peanut allergy?

A: In short, the answer to this is "yes." But the answer to this requires consideration of the unpredictability of a subsequent reaction. There are people who may have ten reactions over their lifetime and maybe one of the reactions would be "severe." Because reactions may vary from time to time, we often think of peanut allergy as "potentially severe," even if a person has not experienced a severe reaction.

Q: How often is a severe reaction to peanut fatal?

A: Surprisingly, there are no studies that have addressed this question directly. However, it is estimated that in the United States, approximately 100 to 150 people die each year from a peanut allergy.

Q: It appears that peanut allergy is more common now than in the past. Is that true or is there just more public awareness and publicity?

A: If you walk into any school and ask a school nurse who's been working there for more than ten years, "Have you seen an increase in peanut allergy in the children in your school?" nowadays virtually all of them will answer, "Yes."

We also have recent data from our studies in the United States showing that there has been a doubling in the rate of peanut allergy among children within the past five years. Similar studies in the United Kingdom have shown an identical increase. These studies used the same methods to determine the rate of peanut allergy in the general population at five-year intervals. In other words, I believe we are truly seeing an increase in the actual number of cases of people with peanut allergy, particularly children.

Q: Why do you think there has been an increase in the number of peanut-allergic people?
A: There are two general thoughts about why we are seeing an increase. One theory regards allergy in general, which is that many different types of allergy and allergic diseases have increased in the past two decades. For example, over this short time asthma almost doubled, atopic dermatitis, or eczema, an allergic type of skin rash, has doubled or tripled in the last few decades, and hay fever has also doubled. So it may just be a reflection of this general rise in allergy. Other thoughts are that there are peanut-specific reasons why there has been an increase in this allergy.

Q: What are some of these peanut-specific causes for an increase?
A: In regard to peanut allergy in particular, there is a theory that roasting peanut, which is what is done for making peanut butter, makes peanut proteins more likely to cause allergy. Westernized societies commonly use roasted peanut products (see below for further explanation). Another theory is that we often introduce peanut very early into the diet of children who may be susceptible to peanut allergy, and that could be another reason for an increase.

Other peanut-specific reasons have been brought up in studies from England showing that using topical moisturizing ointments containing peanut protein on the skin for treating children with dry skin or allergic skin rashes has been associated with increased peanut allergy. In that same study, feeding soy formula was also associated with increased peanut allergy. Interestingly, if mothers used peanut-containing nipple creams while breast-feeding, that was not a risk for peanut allergy. It should be noted that nipple creams or skin creams that contain peanut protein are not widely used in the United States, so it would be very difficult to blame these types of creams for the rise in peanut allergy in the United States.

Q: What do you think accounts for the difference between the peanut-containing nipple creams not being associated with peanut allergy versus the peanut-containing skin creams used on the babies that were associated with peanut allergy?

A: One of the theories about this is that when the babies get oral or mouth exposure to peanut protein, the body may not react in the same way as when the same exact protein is used to coat their skin that is already inflamed with allergic skin rashes. In other words, the immune system may respond more normally to food in the mouth as opposed to food rubbed all over the skin. However, more studies are needed to sort this out.

Q: Why is peanut used in these creams to begin with?

A: The peanut oil is used as a moisturizing component. Some oils contain peanut proteins, and some do not. In any case, there are numerous good moisturizers that have no peanut oil.

Q: Returning to the possible problem of roasted peanuts, why would they cause more allergies?

A: It's been observed that there is less peanut allergy in China, for example, yet they ingest about the same per capita amount of peanut as we do in the United States. However, they fry or boil their peanuts, whereas in the United States and other westernized countries, we roast them. So it is possible that the type of heating process actually changes the proteins in peanut in a way that makes our immune system more likely to react to them, or that they get from our gut into our bloodstream more easily. To summarize this issue: roasting peanuts may create a more allergic type of peanut than boiling or frying peanuts.

Q: Is the way we eat peanuts now different from the way we ate them a few years ago?

A: That question actually points out the weakness in the theory that the way that we're eating peanut accounts for the increase in peanut allergy in regard to roasting them or the age at which they are eaten by children. In other words, there are no verified studies showing that we're eating more peanuts now, or that we're giving peanuts to our children at a younger age, or that we're roasting them differently now than we did five or ten years ago. So in a sense, this is a question that points out a weakness in the theory that it's specifically how we're treating our peanuts that has caused the rise in peanut allergies.

Q: What is the relationship between rashes in infants and peanut allergy?

A: In a study from England, one of the associations found that babies who had allergic types of skin rashes were more likely to have peanut allergy. I would interpret that finding primarily to reflect that babies with allergic skin rashes are generally prone to allergy, and so they're also more prone to have allergic diseases like asthma and more likely to have food allergies in general. So it's not necessarily a cause-and-effect relationship but one that just reflects an increased disposition to develop an allergy to anything, including peanut.

Q: How do you explain the relationship between the use of soy formula and peanut allergy?
A: A British study showed that if babies used a soy formula, they were at a bit over double the risk for developing a peanut allergy compared to infants who were not fed soy formula. Scientists who have reviewed this study have asked a very simple question, which is, perhaps it isn't really a cause-and-effect relationship with the soy formula, because babies with eczema so often have their formulas switched. But the people who did the study believe they adjusted for that possibility, so there's some controversy about how strongly the use of soy formula can be associated with peanut allergy.

However, the reason that there could be a relationship is that soy is a bean, and peanut is a bean. So if the infants became allergic to soy formula, there may have been some carryover to another bean, namely peanut. The complicated issue here is that none of the infants in that study had both a soy allergy and a peanut allergy, and you would have expected that they would have had both if there were really a relationship.

So a great deal more study is necessary in order to determine whether soy formula is actually a risk for peanut allergy. The current American Academy of Pediatrics' guidelines for prevention or delay of food allergy does not recommend soy as a hypoallergenic formula in the first year of life. If those recommendations were followed, this would not be a specific issue.

Q: What other theories do people have for the rise in peanut allergy, if it is not due solely to the use of peanut itself?
A: It goes back to the idea that there is just a general increase in allergic disease, and peanut is a part of the reflection of the increased rise of such conditions as asthma, allergic skin rashes, and hay fever, as well as other food allergies. This all goes to a theory called the "hygiene hypothesis," or "cleanliness hypothesis."

It has been found that people who live in less clean environments, for example, those who live on farms or who have multiple animals in their home, or who have grown up with older siblings from whom they might have caught colds, or who have not been treated that much with antibiotics, or live in countries where vaccination has not been used liberally, all have lower rates of allergic diseases compared to the converse situation.

Q: Why would people living in less clean environments have fewer allergies?
A: The idea here is that if the body's immune system is not being kept busy fighting bacteria or other germs, then the immune system is left unoccupied and may attack otherwise harmless proteins in the environment. For example, the immune system may respond to pollens and animal

dander, resulting in asthma or hay fever, or in the case of peanut allergy, the proteins in this common food.

The other interesting thing about our immune system that ties in with the hygiene theory of allergy is that the part of the immune system that creates allergies is also the part of the immune system that fights parasite infections. We're living in an industrialized society where we're not really exposed to parasites, so our immune system does not have that aspect of infection to keep itself busy and can therefore turn that arm of the immune system against otherwise harmless proteins like peanut.

Q: Would it be better not to vaccinate our children or not to use antibiotics?
A: That certainly would not be a good strategy! Vaccination, antibiotics, and sanitation have prevented many more deaths and illnesses than ever occur from allergies. It may be that exposure to some "good germs" may activate a healthier immune system that is less likely to attack harmless proteins (for example, as may occur with farm living). So the issue here is more one of asking if there are other things we can do to help ourselves to avoid allergic disease, despite the fact that we want to use treatments such as vaccination and medications to prevent ourselves from suffering or dying from other causes.

Q: So not all germs are bad?
A: It is a very tricky and complicated balance. Some germs make us sick, and others do not. Some studies have shown that the types of bacteria we are exposed to may influence allergy outcomes.

Q: Is there a way we can get good germs into our bodies?
A: There actually may be a way to get "good" germs, or possibly the chemicals in those germs, that direct "healthy" immune responses, and this is one active area of research. For example, the study of probiotics, bacteria that may promote "healthy" immune responses, shows some promise. However, their efficacy for prevention or treatment of peanut allergy is not known at this point, and studies on allergic disease have so far been few.

3

Who Develops Peanut Allergy and Some Reasons Why

Q: Why does one person develop a peanut allergy, while another person doesn't?
A: Those of us who have studied peanut allergies really believe that they are a result of both environmental and genetic, or hereditary, influences. In fact, peanut allergy is more likely to occur in people who have allergic responses, including asthma; allergic skin diseases, such as eczema; and hay fever. The predisposition of the body to make this type of immune attack is probably why some people get peanut allergies and others do not.

There may also be specific things about people's immune systems that make them more prone to developing peanut allergies, in that their immune systems are poised to easily recognize the proteins in peanut, as opposed to some other food or some other item in the environment.

Q: Are you saying that some people are more at risk for peanut allergy?

A: Definitely. Peanut allergy is more common when there is a family history of allergy in general, or peanut allergy, in particular. So, for example, if there is one parent who has asthma or hay fever, their child is more likely to have a food allergy, including peanut allergy. If *both* parents have these allergic problems, then there is an even greater risk that a child may have an allergy, such as peanut allergy. In regard to siblings, we did a study showing that there is a 7 percent risk, or about a ten times higher risk than normal, for developing a peanut allergy if one sibling has a peanut allergy.

Q: Does that mean that everyone with a peanut allergy has some other allergy or relative with allergic problems, or is it just more likely?
A: I would have to say more likely. People with peanut allergies don't necessarily have a family history of allergy problems, food allergy, or peanut allergy. Technically, they have to have a genetically directed disposition, but they may not have a family history.

Q: At what age do people usually develop a peanut allergy?
A: Most typically, it seems to occur during early childhood, around the time when peanut would usually be introduced into the diet. However, it is possible to develop a peanut allergy at any time in life, even as an adult and even when one is elderly.

Q: If people don't like peanuts or get an upset stomach from peanut butter, can that be a sign of peanut allergy?
A: There are many different adverse reactions that people

can experience from foods, such as intolerances, food poisoning, or even distaste, but if the immune system is not involved, it is not an allergy. So if you have someone who feels ill from peanut because perhaps it's just a very fatty food and it gives them an upset stomach, that would not be considered an allergy. You will see in the next chapter what the symptoms of a peanut allergy are and how you can recognize them. But it is also sometimes the case that people who have an aversion to peanut may turn out to be allergic.

4.

The Symptoms and Severity of a Peanut Allergy

Q: What are some of the most common symptoms experienced by a person with a peanut allergy?
A: Typically, reactions from peanut can affect any of a number of areas of the body, including the skin, lungs (breathing), gut, and possibly even the heart. The reactions or symptoms usually occur minutes after the peanut has been ingested.

Q: What are the typical symptoms affecting the skin?
A: The most common skin symptoms from peanut allergy are hives, which look like mosquito bites, small raised areas that are itchy. Hives are also sometimes called wheals, and the medical term for them is *urticaria*. Sometimes an individual will get a large number of hives, and there will be quite a lot of swelling. Another skin symptom is just an itch or a redness to the skin; sometimes people will get blotches. And lastly, there can be swelling of the skin, which doctors call *edema* or *angioedema*. Swelling in the

skin could, for example, make the lips appear very large; or the areas that have rashes can get swollen all out of proportion. Sometimes the face can swell up quite a bit, particularly the eyelids.

Q: What are some of the more common symptoms affecting the lungs or breathing?
A: In terms of the area from the neck up, the nose can get congested or runny; the throat might feel as though it is tightening because of swelling that is occurring there, or with swelling of the tongue; and it may be difficult to get air to go in and out of the throat.

In regard to the lungs, the breathing tubes can get constricted or tighten, making it harder for air to go in and out. That is exactly the same thing that happens during an asthma attack, where there is swelling inside the lung with tightening of the breathing tubes and development of mucus in the lungs, also making it hard for air to go in and out.

Q: What are some of the common symptoms that affect the gut?
A: The typical symptoms for the gut are itchy mouth, stomach pain, nausea, and possibly vomiting and diarrhea. It may be actually a good thing that the stomach wants to expel the proteins that are causing a problem, but it could also be dangerous, because you can potentially choke on vomit or inhale it and damage the lungs.

Q: How can you tell if the heart is affected?
A: One of the most dangerous aspects of an allergic reac-

tion to peanut would be if the circulation is affected, which would mean that the heart is not pumping adequately, and the blood vessels may get floppy or dilate, making it harder to get blood to circulate throughout the body, and blood pressure drops. This state of poor circulation is called shock. In shock, the symptoms you might see include paleness, dizziness, disorientation, and loss of consciousness. The pulse may be weak. In addition, some individuals will also describe a feeling of impending doom, even before anything happens.

Q: In addition to these common symptoms, are there any other symptoms people with peanut allergy may experience?
A: Women may experience uterine contractions. People also describe a tingling feeling in the mouth or a funny or metallic taste in the mouth; others have a feeling of flushing. And again, some have that strange feeling of impending doom.

Q: What is the typical time lapse between ingestion of peanut and actually having an allergic reaction?
A: About 80 percent of the time, these symptoms will occur within twenty minutes of an ingestion. But it is actually quite common for them to happen within five minutes. The progression of the reaction could be anywhere from very quick—within minutes—to over hours. And no one knows why it varies that way.

Q: What is anaphylaxis?
A: Unfortunately, there is no universal, simple definition of anaphylaxis. In simple terms, the word refers to a se-

vere allergic reaction. Anaphylaxis is technically described by doctors as an IgE antibody–triggered reaction, where there is a generalized allergic reaction. It is a reaction where the symptoms happen away from where the trigger was.

For example, if you eat peanut, and it's in your stomach, and you get a hive on your pinkie finger, that technically would be anaphylaxis. However, the hive on your pinkie would intrinsically not be a dangerous problem. And anaphylaxis usually connotes a severe allergic reaction. When most people describe anaphylaxis, the emphasis is that it is a generalized allergic reaction, usually affecting more than one part of the body, and it is or can become life-threatening. A person with anaphylaxis may have trouble breathing or have circulatory problems that potentially are life-threatening.

Q: So when you use the term anaphylaxis, you are referring to a severe allergic reaction?
A: That's right. The term "anaphylaxis" will be used in the rest of this book to mean a severe allergic reaction.

Q: Does the reaction get worse each time it occurs?
A: It's actually a common myth that reactions to peanut will be worse with each subsequent exposure. The truth is that a reaction will not automatically be more severe from one time to the next. In some regard, a reaction is more likely to be similar from one time to the next. But it's not even that simple. The unpleasant reality is that allergic reactions to peanut are *unpredictable* from occurrence to occurrence. The same individual might have a mild reaction

one time, a severe reaction the next, a mild one after that, and then a severe one again, with no specific rhyme or reason that we have been able to find.

In one study we found that for children over the age of four years, their reaction from time to time was roughly similar. However, we also did a study looking at very young children with peanut allergy over a period of time as they got older, from approximately the age of one to ten years, and there was a slight increase in the severity of reactions from when they were very young children to the time when they were older children. We believe that the increased severity over time is explained by two factors. First, as the children get older, they are more able to describe some of the symptoms that might make us consider a reaction to be severe, such as "My throat is feeling tight." A one-and-a-half-year-old cannot say, "My throat is tight," whereas a six-year-old can. Also, having asthma increases the risk of a severe reaction and more of the older, compared to the younger, children had developed asthma.

Q: So the symptoms may be unpredictable, but that also means that they won't necessarily get worse each time?
A: That's right. They won't necessarily get worse, but they might. The fact that a first reaction was mild does not preclude the possibility that a subsequent reaction could be severe or life-threatening.

Q: Does it matter how much peanut you have eaten in regard to the severity of the reaction?
A: That is a difficult question because the more you eat, presumably, the more severe the reaction would be. How-

ever, even a small amount could potentially trigger a reaction, including a severe one.

Q: So the answer to the question about the severity of the next reaction has to be, "We don't know"?
A: Yes. The answer is that a reaction could vary in the same person over time, it can vary despite a particular amount eaten, and so again, it's unpredictable. And there is simply not a stable relationship or an exact correlation between the severity of an allergic reaction and the amount of peanut that is eaten or the number or severity of previous reactions.

Q: How do you know if you have a very severe peanut allergy?
A: Unfortunately, you usually don't. That is because most people who have had a peanut-allergic reaction will not have had an extremely severe reaction. The unfortunate people who have died from an allergic reaction to peanut did not typically have a history of numerous previous severe reactions.

But if you have had a severe reaction to peanut previously, then you certainly know that you could potentially have one again. If you have never had a severe reaction to peanut, there is no specific test that can tell you that you have a severe peanut allergy. But because we know that reactions may vary from time to time, and it's always possible to have a more severe reaction, we will teach people to assume that their peanut allergy could be severe.

Q: Can you define a person who is "at risk" for a severe peanut allergy?

A: If you have a peanut allergy and have had previous severe reactions, you are clearly at risk for another severe reaction in the future. The other key factor is *underlying asthma*. In many different studies, having underlying asthma is a risk factor for a more severe reaction if you ingest peanut and have peanut allergy.

Q: Could it be fatal if you have asthma and a peanut allergy and eat peanut?
A: Unfortunately, it *can* be fatal. Although there are not many studies on the epidemiology of fatal reactions to peanut, it seems from the available studies that peanut is one of the most common causes of food-induced fatal allergic reactions.

Q: Is there any way to predict if a peanut-allergic reaction will be fatal?
A: There is no specific test that can determine if you have a risk for a fatal peanut allergy. However, there is a crucially important theme we have learned from studies where a food allergic reaction was, unfortunately, fatal. Persons who have had fatal reactions from peanut tend to be *teenagers or young adults with asthma and a known peanut allergy who did not promptly receive their emergency medication when they had a peanut reaction. In addition, fatalities more typically occur when eating outside the home.*

This theme of a teenager or young adult being at risk for a fatal reaction to peanut probably reflects the fact that teenagers are more likely to assume risky behaviors. For example, they are more likely to eat foods that are riskier in regard to containing peanut. And teenagers are also classically known to deny symptoms, so if they're having throat-tightening or other symptoms that would indicate "You should be using your medication," they are more likely to say, "I'm just going to sit this one out and maybe go to my room alone and hope it will pass." It's that exact combination of risk-taking and denial of symptoms that we believe results in this particular age group being at highest risk for a fatal reaction.

Q: What about the teenagers not using their medications? Why didn't they use them?
A: They either didn't have the medications with them, or they simply decided not to use them. They may also inappropriately try to treat their severe allergic reactions with the wrong medication, such as using an asthma inhaler when they should be using self-injectable epinephrine (as described in chapter 13). Unfortunately, many teenagers have a tendency to think they are immortal and nothing can happen to them. Of course, now that this issue is known, it is a goal to make all necessary efforts to educate teenagers about their allergies and enlist their friends and others to insure their safety.

Case History

DORA

Dora, the thirty-seven-year-old mother of one of my peanut-allergic patients, came to see me to find out if she was also allergic to peanuts and if so, whether or not she could have a severe allergy. Dora told me that she had a lifetime history of mild reactions to peanuts, she did not really like their taste, and generally avoided them. On the dozen or so occasions when she had eaten peanuts, she experienced a very itchy mouth and throat, and a few times her lips also swelled. Although she had eaten up to twenty peanuts at a time, her symptoms had never gone beyond her mouth and lips.

After talking to Dora, I discovered that she also experienced an itchy mouth when she ate peaches and apples, but not every time. She also told me that she had hay fever when birch trees were pollinating.

The information about the birch trees was significant, because there are certain proteins in birch pollen, in some rock fruits like apple, peach, and plum, and in peanut that look alike to the immune system. For some people who are allergic to birch pollen, certain of these related fruits also cause mild allergic symptoms. These allergic reactions are usually to the raw fruit, and when it is cooked, as in a baked apple or peaches in a pie, there is usually no reaction. Dora confirmed that she did not have any allergic reactions to cooked fruit.

I told Dora that most of the time, people who experience these mild symptoms to fruits never have serious allergic reactions, although a small minority can have such reactions or may develop them later on. It seemed possible that Dora was allergic to the protein in peanut that was related to the protein in the fruits and birch pollen.

Dora underwent allergy tests, and we found that she had positive skin tests to peanut, birch pollen, and raw forms of the fruits. But was she at risk for a severe peanut allergy? Although Dora had experienced about a dozen reactions without any severe symptoms, indicating that she might not have a severe allergy to peanut, there is no simple test to verify that Dora would never have a more severe reaction. In studies of people with birch pollen–associated peanut allergies like Dora, twelve out of twenty adults had severe reactions to peanut.

Since these studies indicate that Dora might indeed be at risk of a severe peanut allergy, we agreed that given the fact that she didn't like peanut anyway, she would avoid eating it and would also have an emergency action plan, including self-injectable epinephrine, a lifesaving medication for a severe allergic reaction, just in case she ever had more serious symptoms from an accidental exposure.

5.

Understanding Peanut-Allergic Reactions

Q: Can you review the common symptoms of a peanut-allergic reaction and anaphylaxis?
A: The symptoms can affect any of several areas of the body, including:

• The skin, with swelling or hives or itchiness and flushing;

• The gut, with pain, vomiting, nausea, diarrhea;

• The airways above the neck, with nasal symptoms, like stuffy nose or runny nose;

• The throat, with throat-tightening;

• The lungs, with asthmalike symptoms of wheezing and cough, trouble getting air in and out; and

• The circulatory system, where the heart doesn't function well, and the blood pressure drops. This could lead to symptoms such as paleness, weak pulse, loss of consciousness, and potentially, even death. And this is what essentially defines anaphylactic shock.

Q: Which symptoms are dangerous?
A: The intrinsically dangerous symptoms are:

• Trouble breathing; and

• Poor circulation.

It is not dangerous to have hives, but the issue is always what could happen next.

Q: How do you know what will happen next?
A: Unfortunately, you don't. The problem is that there are many people who may have just hives from an allergic reaction, but essentially, it is not predictable whether or not if one moment you have hives, you're then going to go on to have more than just hives. So, ultimately, you don't really know what's going to happen next.

Q: How long after eating peanut does a symptom usually start?
A: Most commonly, the symptoms will occur within minutes of ingesting peanut. However, there can be a delay, and sometimes the symptoms may not start for an hour or two or, extremely rarely, beyond that time point. But we would almost never expect a reaction to start more than three or four hours after peanut was ingested.

Q: How long may a symptom last?
A: Usually, with treatment, the symptoms don't last more than an hour or two. However, there are situations where severe symptoms can actually recur or last longer, even for hours or sometimes, in rare circumstances, for days.

Q: How can you tell what very young children are feeling?
A: That is a very difficult issue in trying to determine what's happening, because adults can say, "My throat feels really tight," but children can't.

But you may see some subtle things in young children. For example, if they're having problems with swallowing, you might notice that they're drooling. Or if their mouths are very itchy, they may make clucking noises or they may be moving their mouths in a way to use their tongues to scratch the upper part of their mouths, or palates. They may scratch at their ears because when the mouth is itchy, the inside of the ears may also become itchy.

In a significant allergic reaction, children will typically become quiet, because they are not feeling well. And you might notice a sudden change in behavior such as this as a sign that something isn't right.

6

Other Related Allergies: Legumes, Nuts, and Seeds

Q: What other foods are peanuts related to?
A: Although it has the word "nut" in it, the peanut is not a nut. It's actually a bean or a legume, so it is related to foods like string beans, peas, lentils, black beans, and navy beans. The peanut is a warm-season vine plant that actually grows underground, so peanuts are not really related to tree nuts. Tree nuts, such as walnut, hazel, macadamia, and Brazil nut, are nuts that grow on trees.

Q: If a peanut is a bean, does someone with a peanut allergy have to worry about allergy to other beans?
A: Unfortunately, the answer to this is "yes," but fortunately, most of the time, it's not a problem. In a variety of studies that have been carried out concerning this question, we find that about 5 percent of children who have a peanut allergy react to other beans; or conversely, 95 percent of the time, someone with a peanut allergy is perfectly fine with other beans. One of the most allergenic of the beans is

the *soybean*, and soy is one of the most common foods to cause an allergy. And yet, 95 percent of people with a peanut allergy have no problem even with soy.

Q: Do the 5 percent who are allergic to other beans have serious problems?
A: That is quite possible. If someone is allergic and reactive to some of the other beans, such as string beans, soy, or peas, their chances of reacting to multiple beans also increases, so it may be that they're multiple-bean allergic, and sometimes reactions are severe.

Q: Are any beans especially problematic for people with peanut allergy?
A: There are not many studies on this question for children in the United States. Certainly soy is considered an allergenic bean yet, as mentioned before, it is only a problem for 5 percent of children with peanut allergy and even then, most children outgrow their soy allergy. There are studies from other countries that highlight different beans. There's a bean that many people are not even aware of, called lupine. In studies of people with peanut allergy done in France, about half of the individuals who were allergic to peanut reacted to the lupine bean, as well. Presumably, there's some kind of similarity that is stronger between the two, although this relationship has not been completely studied yet. Lupine doesn't show up in too many foods in the United States, but you would be able to find it on the gourmet shelves or on some of the ethnic shelves in the supermarket. Lupine is also used to make bread products (lupine flour.) Chickpeas and lentils seem to be allergenic

beans for people living in Mediterranean countries, but we don't have a lot of information on that in the United States because they are not eaten as commonly here.

Q: If beans such as lupine, chickpeas, and lentils are a problem for peanut-allergic people in other countries, what do you advise your patients here in the United States?
A: I tell my patients about lupine, in particular, because of the especially high rate of a problem. Overall, however, I still emphasize that more than 95 percent of individuals with peanut allergies tolerate all of the other beans, including soy.

Q: We know you can be tested for peanut allergy (see part 2), but is it possible to be tested for allergies to the other beans you mentioned?
A: You can, but it is a bit tricky to interpret the results. If you have someone with a peanut allergy, and you test them with an allergy test for any of the other beans, there's a 50 percent chance that there will be a positive reaction to those beans because they share a lot of the proteins that are in peanut. However, even though about half of the time you'll see a positive test, still 95 percent of the time there is no reaction when they actually eat those other beans.

Q: What if you get a positive test to the beans, but you have never eaten them?
A: If you have someone who is already eating these beans, I would not even test them because you're likely to see a

positive, and it's completely irrelevant. But if they have not tried a specific bean and we are not sure if they would react to it, and we test them and get a positive result, then you usually need to watch them eat the bean under a doctor's supervision to be sure that it's safe. (See chapter 11 for details about these "oral food challenge" tests.)

Q: Even though a peanut is not a nut, do people with peanut allergy have to be careful about eating various kinds of nuts?
A: It turns out that there are not many similarities between the proteins in tree nuts and the proteins in peanut, but to some extent, they behave similarly among people with allergies. That is, nut allergy is quite common and potentially severe, so it's possible for someone who is prone toward food allergy and peanut allergy to also have an allergy to tree nuts.

In fact, in our studies, around a third of peanut-allergic individuals have or eventually develop an allergic reaction to at least one of the tree nuts. Again, that is not because they are related foods but because they are allergenic foods.

Q: Do you do allergy tests for nuts in people allergic to peanut?
A: If they have not eaten the nut and they don't know if they are allergic to it, I will usually test them to it just to find whether there's any risk at all. If they are already eating nuts from trees, there would not be a specific reason to test what they are already eating and tolerating.

Q: What advice do you give your patients about tree nuts?
A: If my patients are young children and have not eaten the tree nuts, even if the tests to them are negative, I'll usually have them avoid tree nuts for several reasons. One reason is that a lot of the products you buy that have tree nuts in them can easily end up accidentally or sometimes purposely, containing peanut. Peanut is a cheaper substitute for "nutty flavor," so if you buy a walnut brownie in a bakery, there's a chance you're going to end up with peanut in it, either purposely or by accident, because peanuts are used in that facility. If you get a nut ice cream, even if it says it has almonds, I would be concerned that maybe it would contain peanut. So for most of the products that would contain nuts, there is a risk of inclusion of peanut, or cross-contamination with peanut.

Additionally, there is a 30 to 60 percent chance for young children with a peanut allergy to eventually develop a tree nut allergy. Conversely, for people who are already eating tree nuts at the time of their diagnosis of peanut allergy, I do not stop them from eating the nuts if they know that they're getting them in a safe way. In other words, if they're cracking open walnuts and eating them out of the shell, there aren't going to be any peanuts in there, so they could keep eating them in that way.

Q: Do peanut-allergic people have allergic problems with different kinds of seeds?
A: There seems to be an increase in the number of allergies to seeds, such as sesame seeds, and it turns out that there are parts of the sesame seed protein that look a bit like the peanut protein. Most people with peanut allergy do not have a seed allergy or vice versa, but we are looking into

the possibility that there is some cross-reactivity that may be happening.

I treat the seed story in the same way as the nut story, in that if someone has not eaten the seeds before, I might test them and inform them about the risks and potential benefits of going ahead and eating products with seeds in them. If they test positive, then we need to determine through a food challenge (see chapter 11) whether they are really reactive to the seeds or not.

Case History

MARSHA

Marsha was a twelve-year-old girl who had been diagnosed with peanut allergy at the age of two. Her tests showed a strong positive allergy to peanuts, so she had been avoiding not only peanuts but tree nuts as well, since the family knew that as a peanut-allergic person, Marsha had an increased risk of allergy to tree nuts. They also wanted to avoid any possibility of cross-contamination with peanut, so Marsha and her family thought avoiding all nuts was the safest thing to do.

But at the age of twelve, Marsha came to see me because her family continued eating nuts, which were a big part of their snacks, and she felt left out. She knew she could not eat peanut, but she had never been evaluated for tree nut allergies and wanted to know if it was safe for her to eat them with her family.

I explained that most people with peanut allergies do not have problems with tree nuts, since peanut is actually a bean, not a nut. I also discovered that Marsha ate certain other allergenic foods, such as shellfish, without any problems, so she did not seem prone to multiple allergies. Marsha had skin tests for eight different tree nuts and every test came out negative. I told Marsha and her family that a negative test was not a lifetime guarantee that no allergy would ever develop, but that if she was not allergic by age twelve, it was very unlikely that she would develop an allergy to any of these tree nuts in the future.

Just to be safe, I suggested that the family give Marsha nuts directly out of the shell to avoid any possibility of cross-contamination with peanut. By eating them in that way, she would be able to enjoy nuts with her family as often as she liked. Of course, Marsha was very happy with this news and has improved her quality of life by feeling free to enjoy nut snacks with her family.

7

Can Peanut Allergy Be Prevented?

Q: Is it possible to prevent peanut allergy?
A: We would like to find a way to do just that, especially
since in recent years, there has been a clear rise in peanut
allergy. In studies conducted in the United Kingdom over a
five-year period, there was a doubling, and nearly a
tripling, of peanut allergy in young children. In our
population-based studies in the United States between 1997
and 2002, we also saw a doubling, from 1 in 250 to 1 in 125
young children with peanut allergy, using the same study
techniques. Studies of school-aged children in Canada have
documented a rate of peanut allergy a bit over 1 percent.

Among health care professionals and the general public
affected by this problem, there is a very strong wish to prevent peanut allergy, considering that we're seeing such a
dramatic rise in this often severe, potentially deadly allergy. However, as it will soon become clear, there is no
obvious answer to the problem of how to halt the increase
at this point in time.

Q: What are some of the recommendations that have been made to prevent peanut allergy?
A: Certain people are at higher risk than others for peanut allergy or for having children with peanut allergy. The American Academy of Pediatrics has recommended that if there is a family history of allergy in both the mother and father, or in the mother and a child already born to the family, then that mother might consider not ingesting peanut during her third trimester of pregnancy or while she's breast-feeding, and not introduce peanut into the child's diet until three years of age. In other words, they are recommending this for children of families who are prone to allergy.

Although following these recommendations might be helpful, none of these recommendations has been proven to change the course of or prevent peanut allergy. Professional pediatric and allergy societies in other countries have not uniformly made recommendations about altering the parent's or child's diet in regard to peanut allergy because the studies so far have not been clear-cut on this issue. In fact, there are countries where peanut is fed early in life and no increase in peanut allergy has been documented.

However, the major allergy and pediatric organizations generally recommend breast-feeding for families with a history of allergies as a general way to reduce the risks of developing allergies (not just for peanut allergy but for allergic disease in general).

Q: Can eating peanuts during pregnancy or while breast-feeding actually cause a peanut allergy?
A: Although the American Academy of Pediatrics has recommended *not* ingesting peanut during the third trimester of pregnancy or while breast-feeding, this advice has so far

not been validated. There is a study from the United Kingdom showing that mothers who ingested peanut at these times did not have an increased risk of having children with a peanut allergy. So these recommendations are not based on specific studies but just on notions that the immune system may not learn to "attack" peanut if it does not get a chance to "see" peanut.

Families frequently ask my advice in this area. The way I interpret this situation is that we truly do not know the right answer at this point in time, but I advise them of the current recommendations. Considering the scarcity of studies and evolving recommendations, I would encourage readers to discuss prevention strategies with their allergists, because recommendations may change.

At the time of this writing, I have generally advised families of the current recommendations, and if a family is highly motivated to avoid these foods, they may go ahead and do so, even though we're lacking evidence that it works. On the other hand, there are families with children who are peanut-allergic who have put themselves on a "guilt trip" because they think they have caused the allergy, since the mother ingested peanut during pregnancy or breast-feeding. I tell these families that we currently have no evidence to support their feeling guilty at all. As simple counterexamples, we see peanut allergy in children who were bottle-fed and in children born to peanut-allergic mothers who certainly had no peanut in their diets or even in their homes.

Q: Do you think it is important to strictly avoid peanut, or would reduction of exposure work as well if you are trying to prevent the allergy?
A: The issue here is about strict avoidance. In other words,

comparing whether you would reduce the exposure to peanut by eating less of it, compared to trying to avoid it completely. This nuance is actually a very relevant question, and it may be that, in the future, we will discover some "level" of peanut exposure that is safe and promotes tolerating peanut or a particular safe age of introducing it into the diet. But again, unfortunately, we don't have any specific studies to know whether there is a difference in allergy outcomes whether you are strictly avoiding peanuts, reducing them in your diet, or continuing to ingest them as usual. We will just have to wait until more studies on this question are carried out before we have any answers.

Q: At what age is it safe to try peanuts?
A: As indicated before, recommendations from the American Academy of Pediatrics include not giving peanut to a child who is at risk for peanut allergy until after three years of age. Some experts even extend this to age four, but it would always be a question as to whether a given child would react if he or she never had it before. That is, what can one expect the first time peanut is given?

For example, we might have a child who was kept away from peanut because many people in the family have allergies. Then my patient may ask me, "I've never given my child a peanut. Do you think he would react if I gave it to him?" It would be hard to answer that question without more information. If the child had never experienced any allergic problem at all for his first three or four years of life, in that he doesn't have food allergy, eczema, asthma, hay fever, or any other sign of allergy, I would probably guess that he's not likely to react to peanut either (of course, there is still a finite chance of a peanut allergy). On the other hand, if he's gone through his first three or four years of life with multiple other allergic problems, I would be very concerned that he may also have a peanut allergy, and I would be more inclined to test him before having him try peanut.

Q: If a child who may have a risk for peanut allergy has never yet eaten it, would the test be accurate? That is, wouldn't he have had to be exposed to have a positive test?
A: This is an interesting issue because 70 to 80 percent of reactions in children occur on what the family believes is the first known exposure, usually around the age of twelve to eighteen months. That means presumably some level of exposure has occurred, even though people do not think it has. It may be virtually impossible to truly avoid peanut exposure 100 percent. In any case, this observation tells me that if a three-year-old child has not yet tried peanut and has a negative allergy test, it is not likely that he or she is allergic, and I would generally discount the issue of an absence of known exposure.

Q: What is the risk for a person whose sibling has a peanut allergy to develop one, too?
A: From our studies on the hereditary aspects of peanut allergy, we see that 7 percent of the siblings of a peanut-allergic child also have peanut allergy. I consider that a high enough risk to usually recommend that the child be tested before trying peanut. But do not lose sight that the outcome is more likely good: 93 percent of these children would not have a peanut allergy. But I think the 7 percent risk is high enough to warrant testing. It is actually a risk

that is over ten times higher than the risk in the general population.

Q: What if the siblings are already eating peanut? Should they stop and get tested?
A: Absolutely not. If people are already eating peanut with no problems, then, by definition, they are not peanut-allergic, and there would be no reason to test them.

Case History

STEPHEN

Three-year-old Stephen was the younger sibling of Tracy, a girl with a peanut allergy. To protect their daughter, the family did not have peanut in their home, and Stephen had never eaten it. Since Stephen was about to begin child care, his family came to see me in order to find out if he also had a peanut allergy, since he would now be around other children and possibly exposed to peanut.

I told the family that as the sibling of a peanut-allergic child, Stephen had a 7 percent risk of also having a peanut allergy. I asked if he had ever shown any allergic symptoms or had any health problems that might be related to allergy, for example, eczema or asthma, or a reaction to any foods. The family told me there were none, which made it more likely that Stephen did not have a peanut allergy.

I performed a skin test to peanut, which came out negative, as did the tests for tree nuts. I told the family that he had no evidence of a peanut allergy, he did not seem to be an allergic individual, and it was unlikely that he would develop any allergies in the future. Still, the family asked if it was possible that the skin test was a "false negative," since Stephen had never even eaten any peanut. They asked, "Doesn't someone have to be exposed to peanut in order to get a positive test?"

That was a good question! It turns out that 70 to 80 percent of reactions to peanut occur on the first known ingestion of the food. Indeed, we believe some exposure is needed to acquire an allergy, and we believe that most people *have* been exposed to peanut in day-to-day life activities, since peanut is so common. So I explained that the chances were that Stephen could have been exposed somewhere along the line, and by his age, he would have most likely had a positive test if he had a possible peanut allergy. Although there can be no lifetime guarantee of no allergy, this negative test was a good indicator that he did not have and would not develop a peanut allergy.

Getting Help for Your Peanut Allergy

In Part Two, you will find out how to get help for yourself or for someone who may have an allergy to peanut. We will give you suggestions for finding the right doctor, describe what happens on a typical first visit, tell you what information and material to bring to that visit, talk about the different methods allergists use to diagnose peanut allergies, and look at the course of a peanut allergy over a lifetime.

8

When to Seek Treatment

Q: How do I know when to have my child or myself checked for a peanut allergy?
A: One major reason would be if you suspect that you have had an allergic reaction to peanut. (See chapter 4 for symptoms.) For example, if shortly after ingesting peanut, you experience any of the typical symptoms we discussed, such as skin reactions, including hives (which can be very itchy), swelling (often on the face and lips), redness, blotchiness, or even just itching alone; mouth symptoms, such as itching or a swollen tongue; throat symptoms, such as tightening of the throat; breathing problems, such as asthma, trouble breathing, or a congested or runny nose; gut symptoms, such as stomach pain, nausea, severe or significant vomiting, or diarrhea; or cardiovascular symptoms, such as loss of consciousness or dizziness; these would be reasons to get checked.

If the heart and blood vessels become affected, there can be shock, and the symptoms can include paleness, dizziness, loss of consciousness, or a strange feeling of impending doom.

Other symptoms include uterine contractions in women, a metallic taste in the mouth, and flushing.

In addition, if there is a strong family history of allergy—for example, another child in the family already has a peanut allergy—and the child has never eaten peanut, this may be another reason to be evaluated.

Q: So, if anyone has any of the symptoms you mentioned after eating peanuts, they may be allergic?
A: Yes, that's right. And they should definitely seek medical treatment to get a diagnosis, since it could potentially save their lives.

Q: Can you review the time lapse between ingesting peanut and the symptoms?
A: Eighty percent of the time, these allergic reactions occur within twenty minutes of eating peanut, but they can often happen within five minutes. Occasionally, they may occur an hour or more afterward.

Q: When peanut allergy is suspected, who should do the initial evaluation?
A: In many circumstances, it is possible for pediatricians or internists to do an initial evaluation. They should perform a very thorough history to determine whether or not it's important to check for a peanut allergy (or possibly another food allergy or another medical problem), because if you do tests for peanut allergy haphazardly on the general

population, you will see many positive tests that are not associated with any true allergy to peanuts. So a blood test for peanut sensitivity should only be done when, based on the history, there is a serious concern that a peanut allergy may exist.

Q: If a pediatrician or internist finds that a peanut allergy may be causing the symptoms, what should be done next?
A: The more thorough evaluation for peanut allergy should usually be left to an allergist, who is specifically trained to interpret the tests, provide a management plan, and consider other related issues of a peanut allergy diagnosis. When pediatricians or internists find a positive test, they will usually refer their patients to an allergist for further evaluation.

One tricky factor is that there are some cases where a negative test may occur, even though the person has a true peanut allergy. This is particularly an issue for the blood test, where it may be negative about 20 percent of the time, even though the person has a true peanut allergy. This is specifically where a big mistake could be made, unless there is an understanding of this possibility, and that is specifically why it is so important to have an allergist involved.

Q: In other words, when allergists see a negative test, they have the knowledge and experience to know that a peanut allergy is still possible?
A: Exactly. And allergists then have the ability to do a skin test at that point, which is a more sensitive test (see chapter 11 on diagnosis) and pursue other diagnostic measures, if needed.

9

How to Find the Right Doctor

Q: What type of doctor is qualified to treat peanut allergies? Is it necessary to consult a specialist?
A: When you first suspect a peanut allergy, you will probably discuss it with your primary care doctor, usually a pediatrician or family practitioner, if a child is involved, or an internist. Sometimes, an individual's first reaction to peanut is severe, and the person ends up in an emergency room, so the first physician you see in that situation would be an emergency room doctor.

You can receive good care from these doctors, and they should be able to handle the initial diagnosis and treatment. However, only an allergist has special training in the complexities of diagnosing and treating allergic conditions such as a peanut allergy.

So once people have received a diagnosis of peanut allergy or have a strong suspicion that peanut allergy is the cause of symptoms, they should seek out an allergist. It is my opinion that even though a primary care doctor may manage many aspects of a peanut allergy without difficulty, the condition has many aspects that are best handled by a specialist. For that reason, I strongly recommend consulting an allergist for regular treatment of peanut allergy, if at all possible. The allergist and your primary care doctor can then work together to provide you or your child with the best possible care.

Q: Specifically, what does an allergist do that a primary care doctor may not do?
A: An allergist can conduct different tests to confirm the peanut allergy, evaluate for alternative or additional allergic problems, insure that all issues related to the allergy are clearly discussed and understood, and work out a management plan designed specifically for individual patients and their families. In many cases, primary care doctors refer their patients to allergists when a complex condition, such as peanut allergy, is diagnosed or suspected.

Q: When choosing an allergist, what kind of training and background should you look for?
A: An allergist may have been initially trained and board-certified as a pediatrician or an internist or both. After completing this primary training, which usually takes three years, future allergists then complete a two- or three-year fellowship, during which time they receive training in allergies and clinical immunology.

This training is very broad and includes the diagnosis and treatment of all types of allergic diseases, such as asthma, hay fever, drug allergies, and food allergies, as well as immune system disorders. During the fellowship period, the physician cares for patients of all ages, even if their initial training was in pediatrics or internal medicine. Following the successful completion of an approved fellowship (one that is monitored, approved, and accredited), the allergist-immunologist then becomes "board-eligible." The doctor can then take a further regulated examination through the American Board of Allergy and Immunology, and if these exams are passed, the doctor is then "board-certified" in allergy and clinical immunology.

Although these doctors are qualified to treat patients of all ages, some decide to limit their practices to children or adults, according to their initial training.

Q: Can you recommend some of the most effective methods for finding a good allergist?
A: A "good" allergist is not only a well-qualified doctor but also one whom an individual patient trusts and responds to positively, so I see a person's choice of physician as a very personal matter with many "intangible" factors. Given that, I think a good doctor is one who focuses primarily on talking. By that, I mean taking a very thorough history, explaining to you what everything means and what to do to manage the allergy well, and answering all of your questions and concerns.

There are many ways to find a good allergist. Sometimes my patients move away to an area where I don't know any allergists I can recommend. In those situations, I suggest that the family begin by finding a primary care doctor they like and then asking that doctor for a recommendation, since he or she would know the local physicians.

You can also ask any friends or relatives who you know have allergies and are seeing allergists for a recommendation.

Finally, you can do an Internet search. Several organizations allow you to put in a zip code and other search factors in order to generate a list of board-certified allergists in your area. (See the resources section at the end of this book for specifics.)

Q: Is it important to find an allergist who has a lot of experience treating people with peanut allergies?
A: All allergists are trained to diagnose and manage peanut allergy, and they all should be able to do so. However, there are some allergists, like me, whose practices focus more on food allergies and who therefore have some added experience in this specific area.

For instance, not all allergists routinely perform oral food challenges, and if they feel one is necessary for their patient, they may refer the patient to an allergist like me, who often undertakes these procedures. So if it is a concern, you might want to initially ask the allergist about his or her experience with treating peanut allergies.

10

Your First Visit to the Doctor

Q: What should a family do to prepare for the first visit to an allergist?
A: When a family comes to see an allergist—and this can apply to any doctor—they may want to think carefully in advance about exactly what symptoms occurred that led them to this visit. In other words:

• What food(s) were eaten?

• How long did it take after eating the food before there was a reaction?

• What symptoms were observed?

• Had the person ever eaten peanut before?

• How much was eaten?

• What was the peanut in?

• Is it possible that foods other than peanut were eaten and that they may have caused the problem instead of peanut?

• Are you certain there was peanut in the suspected food?

So, for example, if it was a restaurant meal, you may want to talk to the restaurant personnel before coming in for an evaluation, to confirm exactly what was in the food. It might turn out that additional or alternative culprits can be identified. This also applies to any packaged foods that may have been eaten. It's an even better idea to actually bring in the package labels, since the allergist may be able to interpret the ingredients more easily that way.

If you visited the emergency room or their doctor, you should bring copies of the tests and records or arrange to have them sent ahead of time to the allergist. If you have had any other allergy tests done previously, you should also make sure the allergist gets copies.

A diet record can also be helpful, listing everything you have eaten over a three-day period, including the times each food was eaten and what symptoms, if any, were experienced and at what time. For example, sometimes an individual may have eaten peanut on other occasions without a problem, and the allergist will be interested in how often that has happened. Because again, if someone has been eating peanut many times without a problem and then suddenly has a problem, it's more likely that the cause of the problem was something other than peanut.

Q: Is it also a good idea to bring a written list of questions?
A: That is very important, and I am always very pleased to see this happen. People should write down any questions they have, so they can go through them with the allergist during the visit. Often, people who come to see me don't

have a list of questions with them. So I usually say to them, "What questions do you have for me? Let's go through them." Then I go ahead and rhetorically ask and answer other questions on topics I believe they should consider.

Some of these questions include:

- How severe is my peanut allergy?

- Is my allergy going to last forever, and if not, when will it go away?

- Do I need to take medication? How and when?

- What should I do if I have a severe reaction?

- How do I approach eating outside my home?

- How much peanut may cause a reaction for me?

- Can I continue to play sports, attend school, and take vacations?

- Can I eat out in restaurants with my family and friends?

- How can I be sure I don't eat foods with peanuts?

- How do I talk to and teach others about my allergy?

- Can I prevent allergic reactions in the future?

- Are there any new therapies available to me?

And as you read this book, you will become aware of many other questions you may have when you see an allergist. It's always helpful to keep a list and bring it with you to the visit. You can also ask someone in the allergist's office if there is anything the doctor wants you to bring to your first appointment.

Q: Is there anything else an allergist may ask you to do before the first visit?
A: Many allergists ask patients to stop taking antihistamines before the first visit, because they can interfere with allergy skin test results. Different types of antihistamines remain for shorter or longer periods in the body, so the allergist's office may have specific instructions, depending on what antihistamine you are taking.

Q: What if you can't stop taking the antihistamine?
A: If you or your child has to stay on the antihistamine for health reasons, that is fine, and you should *not* stop taking it. You should inform the doctor's office that the antihistamine is needed, and then the allergist can use alternative tests or schedule another visit when it might be possible to go off the antihistamines.

Q: If a peanut allergy is suspected or confirmed, should everyone in the family get tested?
A: Just because one person has a peanut allergy, that does not mean that everyone else in the family also has a peanut allergy. So I would certainly not test anyone in the family who is eating peanuts without any problems, and I would only consider testing people who, for some reason, are not eating peanut or a sibling who was born after the child with peanut allergy, who may be at increased risk.

Q: About how long should a first visit last?
A: Since I believe a good allergist is someone who spends more time talking and answering questions than doing

tests, I find that a first visit for peanut allergy should typically take at least an hour. That's because the doctor needs to ask a lot of questions, listen to a lot of answers, and then give a lot of instructions and review everything. And for people who have a diagnosed peanut allergy, they would possibly benefit from or even require at least one follow-up instructional visit not too long after that first visit, and then routine follow-up visits thereafter.

Q: What typically happens during the first visit to an allergist?
A: On your first visit to an allergist to deal with a possible peanut allergy, the visit will usually start with the doctor taking a careful history, including a general medical history. The allergist will ask you to describe exactly what happened to bring up the issue of a peanut allergy. You will also be asked about any other food allergies and allergic problems you or your child may have and whether other family members have allergies.

The doctor will then perform a physical examination. After that, based upon information available at that point, the allergist may perform some tests, which are described later on in this book (see chapter 11.) They may include allergy skin tests, blood tests, or both.

At that point, if an allergy can be diagnosed, or if there is a tentative diagnosis, the doctor will then have a detailed discussion with the patient or family, if the patient is a child, about how to manage the peanut allergy. Some of the issues discussed, which are also discussed in this book, include:

• Avoidance of peanut,

• Day-to-day issues of living with peanut allergy,

• How to treat reactions, and

• The natural course of the allergy.

Additional factors may also be addressed, including the need for oral food challenge tests and the care of additional allergic problems such as asthma or eczema.

11

Diagnosing Peanut Allergy

Q: Can you give some examples of how you may diagnose peanut allergy in a patient?
A: In some cases, it's very straightforward. For example, a parent comes in and says, "For the first time, my child ate a small bite of peanut butter and within minutes, he had swelling of his lips and face. After we gave him an antihistamine, he was better. Can you tell me if he has a peanut allergy or not?" In a case like this, I would do a skin test, and if it were positive, then the combination of a very clear-cut history of reaction to peanut and the positive skin test would confirm the diagnosis of a peanut allergy.

Other times, it may not be a straightforward diagnosis. For example, another family may come in and say, "My eight-year-old had a dessert that had different kinds of nuts and peanuts in it, and afterward, she had some hives. Do you think she has a peanut allergy?" After questioning the family, I discover that the child has been eating peanut butter for lunch every day. But I also find out that she doesn't usually eat walnuts, and there were walnuts in the dessert.

That being the case, I would probably decide that I didn't need to test her to peanut. What I might expect to find is a positive test to walnut and that walnut was the real culprit.

As a third example, a man comes in and says he ate a peanut butter sandwich and the next day he developed hives that continued for a week, so he wants to know if he has a peanut allergy. But I find out from the history that he had always eaten peanut, even up until that very day, and without any problems. Then I would put together that although hives is a typical peanut allergy symptom, having a whole week of hives a day after peanut is eaten is not a common thing to see with a peanut allergy, because we would expect it to have happened right away and not last that long. So I would suspect that he had a virus or something else that gave him a skin rash, and I would doubt that peanut was the culprit.

As we will see, the history that the patient or family gives me works together with the diagnostic tests to make an accurate diagnosis.

Q: What tests are done to diagnose a peanut allergy?
A: Probably the single most important "test" is the history, or the information that the patient or family tells me about the possible connection between a food and allergic reactions. So although most people would expect me to say that the most important test is some kind of laboratory test, most of the key information actually comes from the history.

Q: Exactly what do you mean when you say "history"?
A: The history refers to details about what happened to the individual in regard to eating peanut and what symptoms occurred, and the general allergic and medical history.

Q: How do you interpret the information prepared in advance by some patients or their families, or what they tell you during the first visit?

A: I am essentially evaluating their story in the context of what I know about food allergy in order to assess if the problem is a food allergy at all, and what the culprit food may be. Are the symptoms typical of allergy? What is the relationship of the timing of symptoms to exposures, and what were those exposures? For instance, if someone told me, "I ate peanut butter and got a headache," I would not consider a headache to be a typical symptom of an allergic reaction, and I would not expect it to be reflective of a peanut-allergic reaction.

And if someone had symptoms that sounded correct for an allergic reaction, but they were not correct timewise— let's say the symptoms were a day after the implicated food was eaten—then again I would start to say that maybe this is not connected.

When symptoms are chronic, they usually are not attributable to peanut allergy. For example, people with chronic asthma or hay fever are unlikely to be chronically symptomatic from a food eaten once in a while, particularly peanut. I would instead suspect airborne allergens, such as pollen or animal danders. In these circumstances, I would have to broaden my thought process to think about other possible triggers.

Q: If a patient comes in and tells you about a reaction but isn't aware that peanuts are involved, how do you make that connection?

A: There are several potential "clues." I have to bring my knowledge of likely causes of a food-allergic reaction and compare them to the history I am hearing about. In regard to peanut, I might be more suspicious if the reaction occurred for someone who does not eat peanut often and ate a food that may have peanut in it, even though the person did not think that it did. For example, peanut can be ingested in a bakery cookie, a salad bar meal, a sauce, or a meal from an Asian restaurant—all food items more likely to contain peanut ingredients on purpose or due to accidental inclusion of peanut during preparation—even though you may not see a peanut in them.

Q: It sounds as though diagnosing peanut allergy requires the skills of a detective.
A: It really does! The doctor's job is to be like Sherlock Holmes and try to put together the clues regarding the meal that was eaten and the timing to the onset of the symptoms. Then there are the symptoms themselves. Do they make sense for an allergic reaction? Was the ingestion of peanut a likely cause? Or was there possibly some other cause? Could another illness be mimicking a peanut allergy?

Another thing that we think about in the history is that it's not that likely to develop a new peanut allergy if you've been eating peanut consistently. So for someone who's been eating peanut butter every day to all of a sudden have an allergic reaction to it is extremely uncommon.

Q: Many people think that it is common to develop an allergy to a food you eat very often. Is that true?
A: No, it is not true. And I think it's a common misconception and that the opposite is more likely true. In the case of

peanut, if you've been eating it regularly without a problem, you are not likely to suddenly develop an allergy to it.

Q: In addition to taking a history of the patient, what other tests are used to diagnose a peanut allergy?
A: We do several types of allergy tests, including skin tests and blood tests.

Q: Can you explain what skin tests are and how they are performed?
A: Skin tests are done using an extract, which is purchased from a company and has a diluted amount of peanut protein in it. The extract is placed on the skin, and then the skin is scratched with a plastic or metal probe that just nicks the surface of the skin. That allows the peanut protein to seep into the skin just a little bit. And in order for the skin test to work properly, the person being tested has to be off antihistamines.

Q: For how long?
A: It depends on the type of antihistamine. If people are going to the doctor and having this type of allergy testing done, before they come to the appointment, they should discuss with the doctor how long they have to be off their medications to allow the skin test to work. Usually, it's between three and fourteen days. This test in which the skin is scratched is called a "prick skin test" or a "scratch test."

Q: How do these skin tests actually work?
A: In the skin are allergy cells, and if you have a potential for peanut allergy, these cells will have IgE antibodies that are able to "see" the protein that was scratched into the skin. So once the protein seeps into the skin, it will be seen by IgE antibodies that detect peanut if the person's immune system makes them, and will tell the allergy cell to release chemicals, for example, histamine. The histamine will then cause the blood vessels to expand, just in that small area, which will give the skin redness. Histamine will also trigger the nerves, which causes itchiness. And it will also make the blood vessels leaky, so you get a swelling. Ultimately, the skin area looks like an itchy, mosquito-bite-looking reaction.

Q: How long does that take?
A: It happens in about ten to fifteen minutes. So the physician gets an answer right away as to whether the patient has made these allergic antibodies or IgE antibodies to peanut with this simple test.

Q: Are the skin tests painful?
A: They are slightly uncomfortable, like a scratch from a fingernail, but not painful. The fear and anxiety of the test is usually more of an issue than pain. We test many children, and the youngest children usually don't cry because they don't realize there is anything to worry about, so anxiety is not an issue for them, and the discomfort is minimal.

Q: What about the older children? Those who have learned to be afraid of doctors, for example?

A: The fear of having someone do a foreign procedure or the anxiety of having to go to a doctor's office is more often seen in the children who are over the age of one year. This group is more likely to be upset by the procedure, but it's really not very painful, and we explain what we are doing and why we are doing it. We also use distractions, such as singing, to ease their anxiety. We emphasize that the test feels like a fingernail scratch, that it's not like a needle or a sting, and the scratch takes just a split second. We also warn them that they may feel itchy, but that goes away soon. If they are uncomfortable afterwards, we may use a cream or antihistamine to ease the itch.

Q: Can a skin test cause a serious allergic reaction?

A: Although it's theoretically possible, it's exceptionally rare and generally not a significant concern. The protein is just at the skin's surface, so we expect only a small reaction at the site of the scratch.

Q: If a patient has had a severe reaction to peanut, is it safe to have skin tests?

A: One of the worries many of my parents bring up is that if I'm touching their child's skin with peanut and scratching it in, could they possibly have a severe or anaphylactic reaction? Based on studies of the safety of skin testing, it's extremely rare to have any reactions beyond the point where the skin is touched with the test material.

So I generally do not worry at all about this issue. On the other hand, if a family is extremely concerned, I don't force them or their children to have the skin test. Instead, I talk with them about the reasons for doing the test. We could certainly do an allergy blood test first, and if that makes the diagnosis, then it may not be necessary to do the skin test.

Q: How is the scratch test interpreted?
A: The test results in a mosquito-bite-looking reaction. We evaluate the size by measuring the bump in the middle, which is called a wheal, and the redness around that bump, which is called a flare. We then compare the results to two other tests. One is a saltwater skin test. No one is allergic to salt water, but sometimes by having the skin scratched, a small bump occurs, so we compare to that negative "control test." We also compare to a positive control test, which is done with histamine, the very same chemical that your body makes in an allergic reaction. The histamine test should be positive.

A positive test to peanut extract only tells you that your body makes the IgE antibodies that are able to see peanut protein. It does not, in and of itself, tell you that you're going to have a reaction if you eat peanut. So that is why the history is such an important factor in the diagnosis.

Q: Are you saying that a person *without* a peanut allergy might have a positive test?
A: Believe it or not, yes, that is correct. We reviewed the National Health and Nutrition Examination Survey data, for which they actually did peanut skin tests in the general population. And it turned out that about one in twenty people on the street has a positive skin test to peanut. That means that they make this allergic antibody to peanut. And

yet we know from other studies that only a very small fraction of those people, probably less than one in ten, would actually be allergic to peanut. So the test is very helpful in identifying these allergic antibodies, but whether a person has a real allergy to peanut is another issue.

To make the diagnosis of a real peanut allergy, you have to put together a suspicion from what's happened to the person together with the test result. It's very strange, even hard to accept, that this is the way to diagnose a peanut allergy. Most people believe a test is supposed to be either "yes" or "no," but it doesn't always work that way. The skin test is excellent at detecting peanut IgE antibodies, so a negative test is very good at saying there is no allergy (though also not perfect), but a positive test does not necessarily give a diagnosis with certainty.

Q: Can you explain how the blood test for peanut allergy works?
A: A blood test for peanut allergy detects the same IgE antibodies directed toward peanut as the skin test does, except it detects them while they're floating around in the bloodstream. A blood sample is taken and sent to a laboratory where it is analyzed to measure the amount of these proteins that are directed toward peanut.

Q: Which test is better: the skin test or the blood test?
A: Both tests are excellent at identifying the peanut IgE antibody. The skin test is a little bit more sensitive, in that if someone has a very tiny amount of these allergic antibodies to peanut, the skin test may be able to find it, and the blood test may miss it. But both tests are quite good.

The distinction is that if the history says there should be a peanut allergy, and the blood test is negative, I would not stop there. I would want to check the skin test, because that test is better at picking up a lower amount of the allergic antibody. Some studies suggest that about 20 percent of people with "undetectable" blood test results but with a history of a reaction to peanut will have an allergic reaction to peanut. Most of these people would have a positive allergy skin test.

Q: What does it mean if you have a positive test but you have never eaten peanut?
A: There are several questions in that question. If you never ate peanut and you have a positive test, you might ask, why was the test done? In other words, was it done because someone had a suspicion that you had a peanut allergy (in which case a positive test is more meaningful), or did you somehow volunteer to have a test done that you really didn't need (in which case the test is less meaningful)?

If you're an allergic person who has for some reason avoided peanut, that would probably increase the odds that the positive test is really relevant. If you're someone who has never had an allergic problem in your life and you're just sitting there with a positive test for reasons that would be hard to explain—someone just decided to do a test on you—then it is less likely to be relevant.

But ultimately, to know whether you would react to peanut—whether you would have an allergic reaction to peanut if you had a positive test and never ate it—you may need to eat peanut under the direct observation of an allergist in order to find out if you will actually react or not.

Q: Would it just be better never to eat peanut for the rest of your life because you're not certain if you have an allergy or not?
A: That would probably *not* be a good idea because you could be needlessly altering your quality of life.

Let's say you just don't like peanuts, and for the last fifteen years you decided, "I don't like them, so I'm not going to eat them." Based on several studies, we also know that if children have an aversion to peanut and just won't eat it, and they have a positive skin test to peanut, half of those children actually do react to peanut when you try to feed it to them. So in that situation, it seems that testing is sensible and informative.

Q: What if the test is positive, and the person has been eating peanut?
A: If you're eating peanut with no symptoms of illness at all, then the test being positive is completely irrelevant, and you should just keep eating peanut. The definition of not being peanut-allergic is that you can eat it without a problem, and if that's what you're doing, then the test is not relevant.

Sometimes an individual has had some screening tests done for some reason, and positive tests, for example to peanut or maybe to some other foods, show up. But if you've truly been eating the food without any sign of a symptom, then that would be a false-positive test. The main lesson is that there is no reason to do allergy tests to foods that are not causing or suspected of causing any problems.

Q: Should such a person have a second test?
A: No. If you are eating peanut and have no symptoms attributable to peanut and were for no clear reason tested to peanut and it was positive, most likely you should forget about it. And as you read further, you're going to see more examples of bad things that can happen if you don't forget about it. In other words, it's probably better to just keep eating peanut.

Q: Can you judge the severity of an allergy from the test result?
A: It would be intuitive to suspect that an increasingly larger skin test size or higher blood level of allergic antibody to peanut would reflect an increasingly severe allergy. Surprisingly, this is not generally the case. One person with a "level 5" may have severe reactions, while another person with the same number may have primarily mild ones. Seeing the numbers go up over time does not necessarily mean that the allergy is becoming worse or more severe (although it may signal that the allergy is persisting rather than remitting).

The tests also do not indicate how much peanut a person can tolerate. The reasons these tests do not reflect these clinical outcomes is probably because there are numerous variables in any given reaction, such as how much was eaten, the person's state of health at the time, what was in the meal that may affect the absorption of peanut protein, and whether or not the individual has asthma.

Q: Can you ever be certain that you have a peanut allergy just based upon tests alone?

A: The more of the allergic antibody you make, the more likely it is that you will have an actual reaction if you ingest peanut. In other words, the blood tests can be measured from undetectable to very high levels of the allergic antibody to peanut. And an allergy skin test could be graded as very small or extremely large. In fact, the allergist scores the skin tests according to size.

For example, the mosquito-bite type of reaction could be either the size of a dime or the size of a half dollar. It turns out that the bigger the test result or the higher the result in the blood test, the more likely it is that you would react. And there are certain levels at which it's actually much more common and almost guaranteed that you will have actual peanut allergy.

For example, in studies in young children with peanut skin tests, if the bump of the skin test is larger than about eight millimeters, there is usually more than a 90 percent chance that they will react to peanut. In regard to the allergy blood tests, several different companies make the tests to detect IgE antibodies to peanut, and so the exact results and way of reporting results varies. One method that has been researched quite a bit is called a CAP-FEIA, UNICAP, or CAP-RAST. The results are reported in units called "kIU/L." The test result is reported from a low of under 0.35 to over 100. Be careful if you look at allergy blood test reports, because different ways of reporting are used, and you need to discuss the meaning of the results with your doctor. However, with this test, about 95 percent of children with levels over 15 kIU/L will have an actual reaction to peanut.

Q: If these allergy tests are somewhat uncertain, how can you find out if you have an allergy or not?
A: If you've had a skin test or blood test to peanut that's indeterminate, meaning that it's positive but not necessarily diagnostically high, and if the history is not a certainty, then an oral food challenge, or feeding the food under the doctor's supervision, is what would be done next.

Q: How is an oral food challenge done?
A: When an allergist is uncertain about whether a person is truly allergic to peanut—for example, if the history is unclear or the test result is unclear—then feeding the food under a doctor's supervision is really the only way to confirm whether the allergy is there. In this test, an allergist feeds a very small amount of peanut to the patient in gradually increasing amounts, usually over a period of one to two hours. Of course, we stop if there are any signs of an allergic reaction.

We begin with a very tiny taste of peanut. The amount is then slowly increased at intervals, usually ten minutes or more between doses. The allergist will ultimately want to be sure that a "meal-sized" amount of peanut was tolerated before declaring there is no allergy.

This test can be done in several ways. Sometimes we will just feed peanut and say, "Here's your peanut butter sandwich. We're going to give you a little bit and then a little bit more." The problem with that is that some people could become very nervous, perhaps even to the point of having a panic response. It's easy to understand that if you have had an allergic reaction to peanut in the past, you would be afraid of someone feeding peanut to you, even under careful medical supervision. Therefore, there is a risk of an erroneous diagnosis of an allergy because of a fear response.

Q: You want to be certain the person's response isn't the result of fear or panic, rather than an allergic response?
A: That's correct. So in order to reduce the chance of a subjective fear response, we could hide the peanut in something else. For example, we could hide peanut in chocolate, using mint, and then feed it so the children or adults are not sure if they're getting peanut or not. This is called "masking" or "blinding."

But when you do it like that, the doctor who is giving the hidden peanut might know that peanut is actually in the food and the doctor might be biased and still overdiagnose. For example, if the person being tested sneezes, the doctor might assume, "Oh, I guess he's reacting to the peanut."

Q: How can that problem of bias be solved?
A: The method that allergists use to reduce any bias in these tests is called the "double-blind, placebo-controlled oral food challenge." It is considered the "gold standard" in diagnosing a peanut allergy. However, it is also much more time-consuming and not always needed.

The way it's done is that peanut is hidden in something else, let's say in a piece of chocolate or in a capsule. And there is also a second piece of chocolate or a capsule that looks or tastes identical but doesn't have any peanut in it. Neither the doctor nor the patient knows which is which, because we have another person make the challenge foods and keep the contents a secret until we are done. And so the patient is being fed gradually increasing amounts of what might actually be peanut or what might not be peanut. However, neither has any preconceived notion of what to expect, and for that reason, it's the fairest way to make the diagnosis.

But a double-blind, placebo-controlled oral food challenge is usually not necessary to diagnose peanut allergy. If an "open," unmasked feeding of peanut is tolerated, or if it results in very obvious symptoms such as hives, using a blinded challenge is not necessary. Equivocal results on such a challenge may indicate that a blinded and placebo-controlled food challenge is needed.

Q: Does this mean that reactions from fear and anxiety can be similar to allergic reactions, and it might be difficult to tell the difference?
A: Absolutely. Later on, when we discuss different treatments, we will give examples of that. Yes, a fear response or a panic response, which really is a normal protective response, and almost an expected one to some degree, may mimic an allergic reaction.

For example, if I point a gun at you, you're going to sweat, you might shake, or you might feel faint. You're not having an allergic response to the gun, but you would be scared by it. So if you experienced a scary reaction to peanut in the past and I am now trying to feed it to you, you may have the same problems, and that is to be expected.

Q: What happens if there is a reaction during this test?
A: If there is a reaction, you stop right away and give medication.

Q: Can it be dangerous in any way to do these food challenges?
A: Under physician supervision, with emergency medications available and with increasing the dose very gradually, an oral food challenge is not considered to be a dangerous procedure. It's been done throughout the world with no reports of fatalities. However, the doctors doing it have to know what they're doing and also have emergency medications available, because it could potentially be dangerous; you could possibly have an anaphylactic reaction. The allergist must make a risk assessment and assure that the procedure is being done in a safe environment. These oral challenges may, for example, be undertaken in the allergist's office or in a hospital, depending upon the assessments of the allergist.

Q: What does a physician do if a reaction occurs?
A: The doctor has emergency medications available during the procedure so that if there are any symptoms, medications can be given promptly. In addition, all of the equipment necessary to reverse an allergic reaction is immediately available.

Q: If patients eat part of the total amount of peanut given and then have symptoms, can they go ahead and eat up to that same amount from then on?
A: The answer to that is "no." For example, if they consumed half a teaspoon of peanut and then started to have symptoms, would it be all right for them to eat up to half a teaspoon of peanut in the future?

The answer to that is "no," because as was mentioned

earlier, a reaction can vary from time to time. And so, the amount eaten that may cause a reaction may be different from time to time. That means that even though you might have tolerated half a teaspoon of peanut this time, maybe you won't tolerate it at some other time. And the severity of the symptoms can also vary from time to time. So we tell people to strictly avoid peanut again if they have a reaction to any of the amounts we use to test them. On the other hand, when we complete a successful food challenge to peanut, we make sure you have eaten a large serving, so there is no worry about eating peanuts in the future.

Case History

JEFFREY

Two-year-old Jeffrey had eaten peanut many times but had never eaten any tree nuts, like almonds, walnuts, or Brazil nuts. When a friendly worker at a bakery gave Jeffrey an almond cookie and he ate it, his face became swollen and hives broke out on his body.

Taken immediately to his pediatrician, Jeffrey was given antihistamines, and his symptoms soon improved. The doctor sent for a blood test for food allergies, which came back positive for peanut but, surprisingly, negative for almond. It was not a peanut cookie, and Jeffrey had eaten peanut frequently and without a problem.

At that point, Jeffrey's pediatrician sent him to see me, since the test results seemed unclear. His parents believed the almond cookie had caused the reaction, and since up to that time Jeffrey had been eating peanut without problems, it didn't seem logical that he was allergic to peanut. Even so, his parents had stopped giving Jeffrey any peanut, since they were now worried he had suddenly developed an allergy to it.

Jeffrey's situation demanded some detective work, since I had to figure out exactly what had caused his allergic reaction, and almond was the prime suspect. Remember that if people eat peanut as a regular part of their diet, it's very unlikely they will suddenly develop an allergy to it, although it is possible. But if Jeffrey's test to almond was negative, then what could have caused the reaction?

My first step was to call the bakery. We discovered that the bakery uses a lot of different types of nuts in their products, including walnut and cashew, and the baker said there could have been walnut and cashew in the almond cookies. I then did a skin test and found that Jeffrey was negative to walnut, but strongly positive to cashew. So I concluded that Jeffrey's allergic reaction was most likely due to an allergy to cashew, which must have been in the cookie, and I told the family that he should now avoid it. I usually have children with one tree nut allergy avoid the whole group of tree nuts for simplicity and increased safety (since the nuts can get mixed up, as happened with this cookie). And because the family was worried about peanut, I also did a skin test to peanut, which yielded only a very small positive response. The skin test was repeated to almond and was negative.

To get a final answer about peanut, I had Jeffrey eat a peanut butter sandwich in front of me. When he had no reaction, I was able to reassure the family that he could safely eat peanut.

I told the family that because of Jeffrey's allergy to cashew, they should be very careful when buying peanut products, to make sure there is no contamination with tree nuts, as happened in the bakery. I suggested they use only commercial, factory-manufactured peanut butter and not buy peanut butter made in small stores, where they sometimes grind cashews or other nuts in the same grinder used to make peanut butter. The family was relieved to know the source of Jeffrey's allergy and felt they could insure that he would not be exposed to cashews.

12

The Course of a Peanut Allergy over a Lifetime

Q: Is peanut allergy permanent?
A: In the past, it was believed that no one would "outgrow" a peanut allergy. That notion was based on studies looking primarily at school-age children or older individuals who had peanut allergy. These studies followed people with peanut allergy over many years and found that none of them outgrew their allergies. However, recent studies have clearly shown that about one in five young children with a peanut allergy actually does not have that allergy anymore by the time he or she is school age.

Q: What are some of the possible signs of outgrowing a peanut allergy?
A: Several of the studies showing that one in five young children can outgrow the allergy also found that the children who outgrow their allergies tend to be those who:

• Do not have a lot of other food allergies,

• Do not have a lot of other allergic problems, and

• Have lower levels of peanut-specific IgE antibodies on their blood tests or have very small or possibly even negative skin tests for peanut.

On the other hand, the severity of the first reaction is not necessarily a predictive factor in terms of who will outgrow the allergy.

Q: When should children be tested for resolution of a peanut allergy?
A: Depending on the family's preferences, we might test them yearly when they are under age four or five. But we are particularly interested in seeing their test results when they are near school age, because of the studies that were mentioned.

However, if an older child has what seems to be a clear-cut peanut allergy, we might still want to test him or her every two or three years, because we have not really investigated what happens to someone over longer periods of time and at older ages. I would not even consider closing the book on an adult who has had a peanut-allergic reaction in regard to outgrowing the allergy, because at this time, there are not any studies looking at that age group.

Q: How would a test show that people have outgrown their allergy?
A: When someone is outgrowing a peanut allergy, we would typically see that the tests are improving. The size of skin tests may become smaller or become completely

negative, or the levels of peanut-specific IgE antibody on the blood tests may go down or even become undetectable.

Q: If the test results are worse, would you exclude any chance of ever outgrowing the allergy?
A: Absolutely not. In fact, it is not that uncommon to see tests for very young children initially go up a bit before going down again. The body's total production of an allergic antibody—not just to peanut but to anything—sometimes increases in the first few years of life. So seeing it go up for peanut is not necessarily a bad sign in terms of outgrowing the allergy.

Q: Does accidental exposure to peanuts make it harder to outgrow the allergy?
A: This question does not have a clear-cut answer. There has been a notion that having accidental exposure to peanut may actually create a situation where it's harder to outgrow the allergy, but there are no specific studies on that point. We looked at IgE antibody levels for individuals for whom we did a doctor-supervised food challenge to peanut and did not see that that exposure caused an increase in the allergy. On the other hand, we did not cause the severe reactions that might happen from larger exposures. So these are somewhat open questions.

Q: Are there any test results that are favorable in terms of expecting the allergy to have gone away?
A: Yes. In fact, there are more and more studies showing that at specific low levels of antibody in the blood, or at

specific small skin test sizes, there is a pretty good chance of outgrowing the allergy. For example, if a skin test is three millimeters—about the size of the word "the" in this book—it's a pretty favorable skin test size for not having an allergy. The blood tests are scored in different ways by the different companies that make them, and only some versions of the tests have been studied extensively. One test, called the CAP-FEIA, UNICAP, or CAP-RAST, measures peanut IgE antibody in "units" called "kIU/L." For that test, studies show that at levels of 2 to 5 or less, about 50 percent of children without a recent peanut allergic reaction tolerate peanut (administered under a doctor's supervision.)

Q: If the tests and reaction history are favorable for outgrowing the allergy, what do you recommend?
A: Living with a peanut allergy has such a huge impact on day-to-day existence that I would be in favor of suggesting that most individuals who have favorable test results and who have not experienced a recent allergic reaction to peanut should go ahead with a doctor-supervised food challenge to determine whether they are really allergic or not. The exact risk assessment for which a family might decide to go ahead with that may vary from family to family.

For example, for a younger child, a family may not be comfortable with a fifty-fifty risk, and they may want the allergist to be able to say to them, "There is only a twenty-five percent chance of a problem." Whereas a family with an older child might be very happy with a fifty-fifty risk or even an 80 percent risk with a 20 percent chance of tolerating the food. So the importance of the food for that family, the impact of avoiding that food on anxiety and social issues for the individual child all have to be considered. If there is at least a good chance to tolerate peanut, the decision as to what to do next is usually made by the family and the doctor together, considering all the different issues that are specific to each person's situation.

Q: Under what situations would you decide to either perform or not perform the oral food challenge to peanut?
A: In most cases, I would almost certainly not do the food challenge if there was a recent reaction to peanut or if the risk of a reaction was high enough—for example, over 80 or 90 percent. However, depending on what the family prefers, I might alter when I would do it. I also would not do an oral food challenge to peanut if the family did not want to actually add the food to the diet.

Sometimes the family might want to see how severe the allergy is by having a doctor-supervised food challenge performed. There are two issues with this. One is, even if the reaction were mild during the time of that food challenge, it would not exclude the possibility that a future reaction could still be severe. In addition, there may actually be an adverse impact on the immune system from having someone ingest peanut just once and then really not adding it to the diet for a long period of time, in that we have seen the allergy return under those circumstances.

Q: So it is possible for an allergy to go away and then return?
A: We never strongly considered the possibility of an allergy returning, because for most foods to which people outgrow an allergy—for example, milk and egg allergies

that are usually outgrown in childhood—we essentially have never seen those come back. And it was not until recently that we started to think that anyone could tolerate peanut if they were ever allergic to it, which led to performing doctor-supervised food challenges. For these reasons, experiences regarding recurrence of a peanut allergy are very recent.

What our research group and others have observed is that among people who completely tolerated more than a peanut butter sandwich worth of peanut butter during a doctor-supervised challenge, some—about 5 to 10 percent—have come back later experiencing reactions to peanut again.

So far, what seems to be common to virtually all of the people who have experienced this recurrence of peanut allergy is that they did not really add the peanut back to their diet. In other words, they tolerated a large serving on that one day we watched them ingest peanut and then decided they were still going to avoid peanut. This experience has also taught us that people with low positive allergy tests to peanut who tolerate eating peanut should probably keep peanut in their diets.

Q: What do you tell people who tolerate peanut during the oral food challenge?
A: For the very reasons just discussed, I tell them to make sure that they continue to eat peanut as if it were a regular part of the diet. We don't know enough yet to tell someone that they have to eat it a certain number of times a week, or how much they need to eat. But I generally instruct them to eat peanut as you normally eat any other food in the diet, the way that most people might eat peanut butter, which is

at least not to restrict it from the diet, and maybe to have the occasional, perhaps weekly, peanut candy or peanut butter sandwich.

Q: What would make you worry about the allergy returning?
A: If a person has really not added peanut to their diet for months after we've done a food challenge, then I would be worried that they may be at risk again, and I may be uncomfortable with them just trying the food again without retesting them. And if a person notices any symptoms in relationship to eating peanut, I would want them to discuss this with their allergist immediately.

Q: When can people stop worrying about the allergy returning?
A: If they have been ingesting peanut as a regular part of their diet for a year of two, I don't have any data saying that we would expect them to have a recurrence of the allergy at this point in time. I generally have my patients continue to carry emergency medications for peanut allergy for a year or two after they have tolerated the food, just to make sure everything is OK.

Case History

JAMIE

At the age of fourteen months, Jamie developed hives all over her body after eating peanut butter. At eighteen months, she was tested by an allergist and had a strong positive skin test to peanut. Her family was instructed to avoid peanut and peanut products, and she had no further reactions.

Jamie came to see me with her family when she was six years old because her family had learned that 20 percent of young children outgrow their peanut allergies, and they wanted to know if Jamie was in that fortunate group. We discussed Jamie's health history, because the fewer the allergic problems, the better the chance of resolution of peanut allergy. I found that she tolerated many classically allergenic foods, like seafood, without any problems. However, she had mild asthma.

Jamie's skin test was a small positive, about the size of an "o" in this book, and her blood test was a low positive (2 kIU/L). These results meant that Jamie had a slightly better than 50 percent chance to tolerate peanut. But the only way to find out was to do a physician-supervised oral food challenge, where we could watch her eat an increasing amount of peanut.

Jamie was nervous about eating peanut, but she wanted to do the test to find out if she could safely eat peanut like the other children she knew. We did the challenge in a hospital, using a double-blind, placebo-controlled oral food challenge, where the peanut was hidden in a food, and the hospital staff, Jamie, and her family did not know which part of the feeding did or did not contain peanut.

Unfortunately, when Jamie ate the food that had the hidden peanut, she broke out in hives and developed a stomachache. We gave her medications, watched her for a few hours, and sent her home when it was safe. Of course, Jamie, her family, and I were all very disappointed that she still had her peanut allergy, but the family was glad they had the information and knew that the measures they took to help Jamie avoid peanut were being undertaken for good reasons.

Part Three

How Peanut Allergy Is Treated

In this section, you will learn about the various treatments for people who have peanut allergy. We will tell you how these treatments work, when you should use various medications, how to understand your symptoms and anaphylaxis, and when you may need to seek advanced care for your condition. We will also talk about various risks of peanut allergy and how important it is for you to clearly understand them.

13

Self-Injectable Epinephrine

Q: What is epinephrine?
A: Epinephrine is a medication that is the first line treatment for a severe allergic reaction or anaphylaxis. It's a medication that opens up the airways so that breathing can take place more easily. It also strengthens the heartbeat and the ability of blood vessels to transport blood to all parts of the body. So ultimately, epinephrine reverses the most severe and life-threatening peanut allergy symptoms in anaphylaxis.

Q: Is epinephrine foolproof?
A: No medication is foolproof. But epinephrine is very good at reversing peanut allergy symptoms and is clearly lifesaving. However, there have been rare circumstances where epinephrine was used, and there were still fatalities.

Q: How do people use epinephrine?
A: If someone is diagnosed with a peanut allergy—and usually when they are, there is a potential for a severe reaction—epinephrine is prescribed in a self-injectable device. In the United States at the time of this writing, the only device available is called an EpiPen. However, other devices are likely to come on the market.

Q: What is the right way to use the self-injectable epinephrine device?
A: First of all, it's essential to review the proper use of this device with your doctor and also to periodically review the use on your own. We did studies on the ability of families to use the device and found that the majority did not use it correctly, and such a misuse could be a tragic problem if an emergency occurred. So I recommend that my patients review how to use the self-injectable epinephrine device on a monthly basis. For example, to make sure you remember, you can do it at the same time that you pay a monthly bill. You need to look at the device, review how to use it, and think about when you would use it.

For the EpiPen device, the gray cap is removed; that "unlocks" the unit. The black tip is pressed firmly into the outer side of the middle of the thigh at a ninety-degree angle and held in place for a count of about ten *without* wiggling the unit. When the unit is removed, the area is massaged, and you should be sure you see that the needle has emerged from the unit. The needle can go through clothing, but I usually advise people to quickly lower their pants so that the needle does not become blocked by the contents of the pockets. The unit can be taken to an emergency room for disposal.

When you hold the unit, it is important not to put your fingers over the ends, just make a fist around the unit. One of the biggest errors we saw in our study was that a parent pressed the narrow end with her thumb, which would have injected the medication into her finger instead of into her child's thigh. Be sure you are holding the unit correctly and are pressing the narrower black tip into the thigh. Afterwards, if you do not see the needle sticking out of the injector unit after you used it, then it did not activate, so try pressing again more firmly.

Q: Are there any videos demonstrating the correct use?
A: The company that makes the device has a Web site that shows a video of how to use it. (See resources.) At this time, there is only one company making the device, but by the time you read this book, there may be others available, so you should check with your doctor on what is best for you.

Q: Is the device dangerous?
A: Although it's rather dramatic to give yourself or your child a shot, epinephrine is not a dangerous medication. Our bodies make epinephrine, or adrenaline, during the classic fight-or-flight response. For example, if something dramatic happens, and your heart beats strongly and you get extra strength to run away from danger, that is due to a burst of adrenaline. In the context of an allergic reaction to peanut, the injection of epinephrine will have very similar effects, but in this case the results are lifesaving, making it easier to breathe and to improve circulation.

Q: Are there any significant side effects or situations where the medication could cause problems, for example, if you are on certain medications or have a heart problem?
A: The usual side effects are the same as those you may experience in the fight-or-flight response. The heart rate may go up, giving a pounding sensation; you may feel jittery; and there can be changes in the body's skin color, such as paleness or pinkness. All of these usually subside in minutes.

These effects are not dangerous for people with normal hearts. However, for people with certain heart problems or the elderly, there could be risks to having the heart race. There are also some heart or blood pressure medications, such as beta-blockers, that interact with the epinephrine and may reduce its efficacy and increase the risks for side effects. If you have heart problems or are taking medications, you should discuss this with your doctor in regard to your emergency use of epinephrine.

Usually, you would be advised to go ahead and take the epinephrine if you need it for life-threatening anaphylaxis, even if you have a heart problem, because the benefit of epinephrine usually would outweigh any risks during a severe reaction. If you are taking beta-blockers or other medications that may interfere with treatment of anaphylaxis, your doctor can often provide an alternative medication that will not interact with the epinephrine. However, in some cases, your doctor may feel that keeping you on a heart medication is more important than concerns about drug interactions from anaphylaxis.

As you can see, these are very individualized decisions that must be made between you and your doctor, and they may vary, depending upon your specific medical circumstances.

Q: Does epinephrine have other uses?
A: It's interesting that this medication was previously used for asthma attacks before inhaled asthma medications were widely available. For example, someone would go to an emergency room or doctor and say, "I'm having trouble breathing; my asthma is kicking up," and they would get a shot of the same drug. Then perhaps twenty minutes later they would say, "I'm feeling tight again; I'm having trouble breathing again," and they would get another shot of it. So several shots can be given, and there is really not much concern about any side effects from it. The main issue is that it will make the heart beat faster and maybe make the person a little bit shaky, but that should not be dangerous for someone who is otherwise healthy.

Q: What if someone took a shot of epinephrine, and it was not really needed?
A: One of the most common questions I get from my patients is, "What if I'm having trouble figuring out if my child needs epinephrine and I don't know what to do?" I always say to err on the side of giving it. There is no significant difference in potential side effects whether or not it was truly needed.

Ultimately, epinephrine is not a dangerous drug. So if you give it and you didn't need to give it, the body is going to behave in the same way, meaning the heart rate might go up, the skin color might be a little different—pale or flushed—and there might be some jitteriness, but it's not likely to cause any damage. So *it's always better to err on the side of giving epinephrine when you're not sure.*

Q: How is epinephrine stored?
A: The self-injection devices have springs, and the drug itself is sensitive to heat and light, so it should:

• Be kept at room temperature;

• Not be refrigerated; and

• Be kept out of direct sunlight and not kept in a place where it can get overheated or frozen, for example, in the glove compartment of a car.

Q: What dose should I be using?
A: Currently, epinephrine comes as two doses. One is a Junior dose (0.15 mg) and the other is a Regular adult dose (0.3 mg.) The manufacturer recommends the Junior size for those who weigh thirty-three to sixty-six pounds and the Regular dose for children or adults who weigh sixty-six pounds or above. However, the manufacturer also acknowledges that the fit is not perfect for persons in between the listed weights and that a doctor may choose to dose according to other factors.

Unfortunately, this dosing availability is not ideal, because obviously, there is a whole range of weights in between, and potentially, there could also be young infants who are perhaps technically too small for even the lower dose. Based upon recent studies, many doctors will switch a person to the Regular-size EpiPen dose before they reach sixty-six pounds. The point where the switch is made is individualized by your doctor based upon the details of your history. For example, the doctor may decide to switch to the Regular dose at a lower weight for those who have had more severe reactions and at a higher weight for those who haven't had more severe reactions and have no asthma.

There is no low dose for infants. Right now, the only other way families can give epinephrine to infants at the usually recommended dose would be to have a syringe and a vial and draw it up in the event of an emergency. Unfortunately, studies looking at the ability of families to do that show that they can potentially make huge errors. Imagine trying to open a vial and draw it up in a needle and give it to your child, who is having an allergic reaction in an emergency situation. It would be very difficult for most people to get it right. This may be a consideration to having a Junior dose prescribed, even for children well under thirty-three pounds.

In summary, I have described some of the factors that an allergist will consider in prescribing epinephrine. But you will have to discuss the right dose and method of supplying injections for your individual situation with your allergist.

Q: How long does the device remain usable?
A: Usually, these devices are good for at least a year. So always check the expiration date right away when you first get it, and then remember to check the expiration date periodically to make sure that it's still good. You can also sign up with the manufacturer for a reminder to update the prescription. The device comes with a small window that you can look into to make sure that the medication is clear, because it can get cloudy or have little visible particles if it has gone bad. The company loads it with a slightly higher strength when they make the device, so that over a year, it maintains at least the label strength.

Although I want my patients to definitely keep an updated device available, I know that studies have looked at the residual amount of drug in expired devices and found, among those where the window showed the drug to be free of particles or discoloration, there was enough residual medication to make use worthwhile if there was absolutely no other available epinephrine.

Q: Who should carry this device?
A: When someone has been diagnosed with a peanut allergy, that usually implies a risk for a severe reaction. As a result, many allergists prescribe an EpiPen for anyone who has a confirmed diagnosis of peanut allergy. There is some debate on this in the medical field. But even though there may be some individuals who have never had a severe reaction and who really seem to have a mild peanut allergy, I tend to err on the side of giving the device to everyone who has a peanut allergy, just in case an emergency arises and they really need it.

Q: When should the device be used?
A: This question seems straightforward, but at times, it can actually be quite complicated. I will attempt to give some general examples, but it is crucial to discuss these issues with your allergist so that your emergency action plan can be personalized. Virtually everyone agrees that if there is a known exposure to peanut in someone who has had anaphylaxis to peanut before, that at any sign of symptoms—and possibly even without symptoms—they should inject epinephrine right away. And the reason for this is that delayed injection of epinephrine can be associated with bad outcomes, including fatalities.

Q: If the allergic reaction is mild, should the device be used?
A: A mild reaction might be defined, for example, as an itchy mouth or just hives that are not intrinsically dangerous. While it is true that many such reactions will never progress to more severe reactions, the decision to use the medication, while it is individualized, should always err on the side of giving it if there's any doubt.

Q: Can you give an example of a situation where you might use the device for a mild reaction?
A: If someone has previously had a severe reaction and he or she has definitely ingested even a small amount of peanut, experts advise giving the medication.

Another example would be an individual who ate a cookie that may have had peanut in it and then immediately started to develop hives. If you know that this person has had a severe reaction before, you would generally be advised to give epinephrine, because it seems that this person indeed had an exposure and a reaction has begun.

Q: Are there circumstances where you might *not* use the device for a mild reaction?
A: Yes. There may be situations where a person with peanut allergy would not get the medication right away. For example, someone who has not eaten a high-risk food and is developing a few hives. If there is no specific reason to suspect that eating peanut is the reason for the hives, and it may be that he or she is having hives for some other reason, you would probably be advised to give an antihistamine and observe the person. In other words, there was no particular suspicion that peanut was

ingested. Of course, any respiratory or circulatory symptom or progression of symptoms would warrant using the epinephrine.

Similarly, people who have asthma may develop an asthma episode from a variety of triggers. Maybe they have a cold or maybe they have been exposed to an animal to which they are allergic. In this case, you wouldn't assume that their asthma symptoms require an EpiPen unless they have had a known or a likely exposure to peanut. Instead, it would seem sensible to have them take their asthma treatment.

I also worry that families may become so allergy-centered that they forget that children can have problems from other causes. For example, if you find your child unconscious at the bottom of a stairway, he or she probably fell, and epinephrine would possibly be harmful. Or if someone had an inability to breathe at all after taking a bite of food, he or she is likely choking and needs a Heimlich maneuver, not epinephrine.

Q: Are there other issues to consider when deciding to use the self-injectable epinephrine?
A: There are many issues that you should discuss with your doctor in regard to influencing decisions about when to self-inject epinephrine, including:

• If you've had a severe reaction before;

• If you have underlying asthma, which increases the risk that you would have a severe reaction if you ingested peanut again;

• If you've had reactions to very small amounts of peanut.

And if you can answer "yes" to any or all of the above three conditions, they are all factors that would argue to be more liberal in using your emergency medications.

Other factors that may influence using the self-injectable epinephrine include:

• The age of the child and ability to judge symptoms,

• The likelihood of exposure to peanut,

• The abilities and qualifications of the person who is witnessing the symptoms, and

• Your location in regard to time until getting medical attention.

Q: Do you need to use more than one dose?
A: Most of the time, one injection of epinephrine will suffice. However, 10 to 20 percent of the time, more than one injection is needed. Therefore, I typically advise my patients to carry at least two units.

Q: How long must you wait between injections?
A: There is no rule here, although people are typically instructed to wait five to twenty minutes between injections, assuming a second injection is needed. But if you've had an injection and your symptoms are getting worse after a few minutes, I would probably not worry about how much time has passed and just use another injection, to be on the safe side.

Q: How long does the medicine last?
A: In one sense, because one injection is usually all that is needed, it lasts "long enough." But the effects of epinephrine will generally wane after about twenty minutes.

Q: How old do you have to be in order to inject yourself?
A: These devices are very easy to use, so even a young child could potentially use one. But even so, I would never expect a young child to be responsible for using it. So it's always a good idea to have other people know about the allergy and also know how to use the medication, especially for younger children and even teenagers, and to have people be responsible for giving it to them. Again, the technique of use is relatively easy, but the decision as to when to use it sometimes also has to be made by someone else. So the answer to this is, it depends on the person.

Q: If you used the device, what else should you do?
A: This is probably the most important question of all, because if you ever have a reaction that you feel needs epinephrine and you give it to yourself or someone else, *you should automatically be going for further care to an emergency room*. The reason is that reaction symptoms can recur in the hours after they began, and when they do, they can potentially be more severe than the initial ones. In a study of fatal reactions to foods, in which several were due to peanut, for many of the fatalities, the course of the reaction included a recurrence of symptoms about an hour and a half after the initial symptoms.

So we generally have people stay in the emergency room for some time, even for four to six hours or more after a reaction, just to make sure that if the symptoms return, help is available. Even four to six hours may not be enough, especially if the symptoms were particularly strong to begin with. So I may have people wait even longer than that for more observation, because you wouldn't want them going home, only to come back. There have been some fatalities reported from premature discharge from the emergency room, when people could not get back in time. In the emergency room, more medications can be given, in addition to the observation. To be clear, using self-injectable epinephrine is not the decision that would lead you to go to an emergency room or not. That is, if you are having a significant reaction and you are concerned about the symptoms, you should go to an emergency room for further evaluation, whether or not you have used the epinephrine (See chapter 17 on advanced care.)

14.

Antihistamines

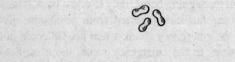

Q: What does an antihistamine do?
A: Antihistamines are medications that block histamine, the chemical that's released from allergy cells during an allergic reaction. By blocking histamine, the effects that this chemical would have on an allergic reaction are also blocked. These reactions include itching, hives, and swelling.

Q: What antihistamines are available?
A: There are a number of different types of antihistamines. Some are available only by prescription and others are over-the-counter. The most common type that you'll find on the drugstore shelves is diphenhydramine, which is available as a liquid, a pill, and a melting tablet that dissolves in your mouth.

There are also newer over-the-counter antihistamines that are a little different because they last longer in the body and are less likely than the older types of antihistamines to make you drowsy. In addition, there are also prescription antihistamines that, similar to the newer ones, last longer in the body and tend not to make you drowsy. But only some of these are typically used in emergency treatment plans for anaphylaxis.

Q: What are the brand names and active ingredients of some of the antihistamines prescribed to treat an allergic reaction?
A: The most common is diphenhydramine (Benadryl) liquid, which is available over-the-counter. Some allergists prescribe liquid cetirizine (Zyrtec), a prescription antihistamine that is less likely to cause drowsiness. There is a large number of antihistamines, but most have not been studied for use in anaphylaxis.

Q: What doses do people commonly use?
A: When used for an allergic reaction, these medications are dosed differently from how they might be dosed for their usual uses, which are for treatment of hay fever or skin rashes. We will typically prescribe diphenhydramine or sometimes one of the other antihistamines for emergency use. The exact doses depend on the individual patient and can only be determined by the physician, but they are generally dosed by the weight or age of the individual. Your doctor can tell you the specific amount that you or your child needs.

Q: Do antihistamines stop a severe allergic reaction?
A: Antihistamines are good at blocking the specific allergic chemical called histamine. However, in many al-

lergic reactions, the horse is already out of the barn, so to speak.

Antihistamines also do not work for some of the most severe symptoms in an allergic reaction, such as the asthma-related symptoms or the circulation-related symptoms. That is why epinephrine is considered the primary medication for a severe allergic reaction. In essence, the antihistamine provides some comfort care and may also help to quell some of the progression of the reaction.

Q: Should antihistamines be used in a pill or liquid form?
A: A liquid formulation is usually recommended to treat allergic reactions, based on the theory that it will be absorbed into the body more quickly than a pill that first has to dissolve in the stomach. Even the liquids can take more than half an hour to really kick in.

Q: Where do antihistamines fit into an emergency action plan?
A: Depending on specifics that you work out with your doctor, use of antihistamines are an additional therapy after epinephrine is given in the context of any severe anaphylactic reactions. Or, depending on what your doctor recommends for you or your child's specific situation, antihistamines may be given as sole medication if there are only mild symptoms from an allergic reaction.

Q: Which should be given first: epinephrine or an antihistamine?
A: This question is usually academic, because they can al-

most be given at the same time. Essentially, any allergic reaction should be treated with antihistamine. The decision issues usually arise on the use of epinephrine. The main issue to this question is that I would never delay giving epinephrine, if it is needed, because of trying to give a child the antihistamine.

Q: What if you are already using an antihistamine and have an allergic reaction?
A: Let's say you are already taking an antihistamine for hay fever. It's OK to take additional antihistamine at the doses recommended for the treatment of an allergic reaction. The slight extra that you take would not likely have any adverse effect, and you may need the additional treatment.

15

Other Treatments for Allergic Reactions

Q: What other medications are used for a peanut-allergic reaction?
A: In the event of a very severe reaction, an emergency room or an ambulance would possibly give you:

• Oxygen to help with breathing problems;

• Intravenous fluids to help circulation;

• Treatments with asthma medications to quell some of the symptoms that are happening at the time of the reaction;

• Steroids, which may be used to prevent the progression of symptoms in the hours after the reaction.

Q: When would asthma rescue medication be used?
A: For people who have a diagnosis of asthma and are carrying medications such as inhalers for their asthma, they could potentially use these medicines at the time of

symptoms during an allergic reaction to peanut. However, an individual has to completely understand that this medication *would not have the same effect as epinephrine*, and that epinephrine is still the primary treatment for any severe symptoms of an allergic reaction.

So, for example, if you eat peanut and develop trouble breathing, you would use your epinephrine first and then use your asthma medications as an additional measure.

Q: Can you provide more information about steroids?

A: Steroids for an allergic reaction are anti-inflammatory medications (not like anabolic steroids, abused by athletes) that reduce a variety of symptoms you may have in an allergic reaction, such as swelling. There is also a theory that steroids may prevent some of the progression of an allergic reaction that can happen during the hours after symptoms begin. However, steroids are usually not part of a general emergency action plan, because they don't take effect right away. As a result, steroids are typically given after an individual has already sought help, for example, in an emergency room.

Q: What about "activated charcoal"?

A: Activated charcoal is a medicine that is usually given in the context of poisoning. It is not the same as charcoal used on a barbecue. It soaks up toxins and could potentially soak up peanut protein from the stomach.

A recent laboratory study looked at the possibility that activated charcoal might be able to soak up peanut protein and, in fact, it did. However, that study was done with peanut and charcoal in a test tube, and there have been no studies looking at the effects of activated charcoal in the event of an individual's actual allergic reaction to peanut. In other words, we need to see the results of a study in which activated charcoal is given to people to swallow in order to see if it inactivates the peanut protein in their stomachs.

Q: Will this kind of study be done? Should the activated charcoal be used in the meantime?
A: There are some concerns about trying to use charcoal in an emergency setting outside of an emergency room. If you vomit charcoal—and it's possible to vomit during an allergic reaction—and then you accidentally inhale any of it, which is called aspiration, it could damage the lungs. Activated charcoal also tastes terrible, and it's not that likely that you would easily get any young people to take enough to absorb the peanut protein that might be in their stomachs. And lastly, it would potentially inactivate other medications that may be taken by mouth, such as the antihistamines. So at this point in time, the use of activated charcoal for treatment of peanut ingestion for people outside of the hospital is not generally recommended. But pending more studies, some doctors might consider it in certain circumstances for people who are already having a reaction and are in the hospital and under medical supervision.

Q: Is there anything else that can be done during an allergic reaction before medical care arrives?
A: There's a recent study of adults having severe anaphylactic reactions that shows that if they were lying down and then were brought up to a standing or sitting position dur-

ing their severe allergic reaction, they got much sicker and some died.

The hypothetical reason for this is that during a severe allergic reaction, blood pressure is low, meaning that the blood has trouble getting to various parts of the body. If you bring somebody upright, gravity pulls their blood down toward their legs. And since during anaphylaxis, the body is already having trouble getting the blood to circulate, having it pool into the legs prevents it from getting to the heart in the first place.

So the theory is that by bringing those who are having a severe allergic reaction to a standing position, you might actually stop their hearts from getting sufficient blood to circulate properly, resulting in a sudden death.

The converse is that when you want to try to improve circulation during anaphylactic shock, you should actually have the victim lying down with his or her legs raised. In this way, gravity pulls the blood from their legs into the rest of their bodies and actually gives them a bit of a boost, so their hearts can have more to work with in terms of getting blood to other important parts of the body.

Q: Is this an accepted practice?
A: Actually, this is a relatively new theory and is also somewhat controversial, especially because we don't know if it is an issue for children at all, and during peanut-induced anaphylaxis, more people have respiratory problems than circulatory problems. We also don't know if there is a risk-to-benefit, because for people who are having trouble breathing, keeping them lying down with their legs up may make it harder for them to breathe deeply compared to if they're sitting up.

Talk to your doctor about this. It may be reasonable that if there are symptoms of poor circulation (poor pulse, paleness, or loss of consciousness), then having victims lie with raised legs is good advice; and it is good advice to keep them in that position while transporting them to the emergency room. For a milder asthma reaction, however, this may not be warranted.

Q: Then the issue of the best body position during an allergic reaction has really not yet been determined?
A: That's right. So it's important to discuss this issue with your doctor and find out what is recommended for you or your child.

16

When to Use Medications

Note: Although we have already discussed the specifics regarding such peanut-allergy medications as epinephrine and antihistamines, this chapter deals with medication in general and knowing when and when not to use it.

Q: What are the primary medications that peanut-allergic people might carry with them, and when should they be used?
A: The primary medications available outside a hospital setting that peanut-allergic people may carry with them are:

• Self-injectable epinephrine;

• An antihistamine; and

• If you have asthma, an asthma inhaler.

A typical question people may have to ask themselves is, "Do I need to use the epinephrine or not?" Because if there's any sign of an allergic reaction, you should always say, "Yes, I'm going to go ahead and take my antihistamine." So most of the problems with decision making center on whether or not epinephrine should be used.

Q: Why is the decision about what medication to use during an allergic reaction sometimes so confusing?
A: The reason that it's sometimes confusing is that when physicians discuss a specific anaphylaxis action plan for your peanut allergy, they need to consider you or your child's specific allergy profile and also the circumstances of a reaction. That means considering such questions as:

• Do you or your child have asthma or not?

• Have you or your child had a severe reaction before or not?

• Who is observing the allergic reaction?

   In other words, parents who are very familiar with their children may be able to make more informed decisions than friends or neighbors who are watching their children, or school nurses may make different decisions than teachers. So there are many nuances in the decision-making process that are specific to the individuals with the allergies and also specific to the situations they are in.

Q: Does the specific type of exposure make a difference?
A: Yes. For example, if you were out at dusk and there were lots of mosquitoes outside, and you were eating an otherwise safe meal and then noticed you had several hives, you would probably simply assume that you just

have some mosquito bites. But if you were indoors eating a lunch that someone else provided and there was a possibility that there was peanut in the food, and then you started to develop itchy bumps, you are more likely to conclude that you may be having a peanut-allergic reaction.

So in the first case, you would certainly not be thinking about emergency treatment with epinephrine, but in the second case, you would.

Q: But if you were outside and made the assumption that your hives were mosquito bites, you could still be wrong?
A: Yes, you could be, but that's the whole point of knowing the history. You could always err on the side of giving epinephrine if you're not sure what to do, because there is little chance of any serious side effects from using epinephrine. But the outcome of *not* giving the epinephrine when you should is far more serious. However, if you know you had mosquito bites and know you did not have peanut, there is no need for epinephrine.

Q: So deciding what to do depends on the specific history of each person and, in the case of children, who is there observing?
A: That's right. Let's say you have a child with asthma who has had a severe peanut allergic reaction in the past and is at a friend's home. The child eats a jelly sandwich at the friend's house and starts to develop hives, but he is a child who sometimes gets hives for no apparent reason. The friend's family has been instructed that if the child has an allergic reaction, he has his EpiPen, and they should help him use it. But should they do it in this situation?

My answer—and I think the answer of most doctors in this case—would be to definitely go ahead and give the epinephrine. The reason is that this child has several clear risk factors that indicate he may be having an allergic reaction that could progress to something more serious than the hives he has right now. Hives are not intrinsically a dangerous symptom. The important question is, could this progress to something more?

Here, you have a child with a history of a previous severe reaction to peanut, which is a risk factor; he also has a history of asthma, which is a risk factor for severe reactions; he's at a friend's home, where they are not necessarily that familiar with his symptoms; yes, he gets occasional hives without a known cause, but this time he just ate a jelly sandwich that they provided, which is actually a high-risk food, because if the family makes peanut butter and jelly sandwiches, they might have contaminated their jelly with peanut butter. So all signs here indicate that an allergic reaction to peanut is occurring in a child who is prone to severe reactions, in circumstances where the supervision might not be adequate. So in this case, I would say the family should definitely give him the EpiPen, even though we are not absolutely certain he was exposed to peanut. Had he experienced his hives and not eaten anything, or had he been with his parents at home, the advice to treat with epinephrine might be different.

Q: Can you give a comparable example where epinephrine use is not clear-cut?
A: Let's consider someone else. She's sixteen years old and has had some very severe allergic reactions to peanut in the past. She's with her friends and is not eating anything at all, but she notices that one of her friends is eating

potato chips. She asks what the ingredients are, and the friend reads the ingredients, which include peanut oil.

At this point, the girl begins to breathe heavily and says she feels like she's having trouble getting air. The question is, should she use her self-injectable epinephrine or not?

One way of looking at this situation is that she has perhaps smelled peanut and, having a history of a severe reaction previously, she is now having trouble with breathing, so that might indicate that she should get the epinephrine.

But another way of looking at it is that she's had some very scary reactions in the past, and her exposure to peanut right now is essentially none, because she hasn't eaten anything, and it's not very likely that she would have a severe reaction from smelling it, especially as a side ingredient in potato chips. So the exposure here, unlike the previous child, is not clear at all, and in fact, it's likely that there is no exposure. The peanut oil may or may not contain peanut protein, and she did not eat it. Her symptom, which in this case is heavy breathing and a feeling of having trouble breathing, could very well be a symptom of anxiety. So the most likely conclusion in this scenario is that she's having some hyperventilation from anxiety about peanut—which is understandable because of her previous severe reactions—but that using the EpiPen would not necessarily be indicated.

Q: Since using epinephrine is not really dangerous, should this girl use it just in case she was somehow exposed to peanut?
A: In fact, I would be in favor of her using it for this particular situation. She is not in a medical setting, she is with her friends, and she is having trouble breathing in association with what she perceives to be an exposure to peanut. Since there is not a specific downside to using epinephrine,

she wouldn't hurt herself if she were to use it. Ultimately, no matter what she chose to do, I strongly recommend that she discuss the entire episode with her doctor, so they can review what the symptoms may or may not have been at the time and so that any future symptoms like these could be judged rationally.

Q: Can you give an example of when epinephrine should definitely not be used?.
A: It's hard to come up with a situation where epinephrine would definitely not be used in the context of an individual with peanut allergy who has potentially eaten peanut, because the risk of using epinephrine is so low in terms of any serious side effects, but the risk of not using it when you think you should is high. There may be a situation where a person has eaten something and isn't sure if it is safe or not. If that person is not having any symptoms, you might want to wait to see if any symptoms develop before using epinephrine.

If symptoms are not associated with an ingestion or have another rational explanation, treatments for asthma (inhaler) or nasal or skin symptoms (an antihistamine) would be appropriate choices. But these are examples where ingestion of peanut is not the main issue. This would be the situation such as asthma from exposure to a cat or from heavy exercise.

But even if an individual with peanut allergy ate something that you definitely know has peanut in it and has no symptoms, but he or she has had serious reactions from peanut before, you should strongly consider giving epinephrine just because the person has such a high risk of proceeding to some type of reaction. And in this circumstance and any circumstances where you are not sure what is occurring or if epinephrine was given, you would go to the emergency room for more observation and possibly more treatment, if needed.

I want to emphasize that in the various examples of treatment, I am not suggesting that there is only or always one "right answer," and you should discuss these issues with your doctor.

Case History

STACY

One day, I received an urgent call from a school nurse concerning Stacy, a six-year-old patient, who had peanut allergy and asthma and had experienced a severe allergic reaction to a small amount of peanut in the past. The nurse was calling because Stacy had come to her complaining of a sudden sore throat. Stacy said that she might have eaten a small bit of her friend's cookie before she felt ill. Her teacher had not been able to determine if she ate any or not, and there was no packaging available for the cookie, so the ingredients were not known.

The nurse said Stacy had a few hives on her face, and she had given Stacy an antihistamine and tried unsuccessfully to reach her parents before calling me. She said that Stacy's throat still hurt, she had a stomachache, she was making throat-clearing noises, and her voice was hoarse. The nurse wanted to know if there was anything else she should do.

It seemed clear to me that Stacy had eaten some cookie with peanut in it and was experiencing an allergic reaction. She had several features of an allergic reaction, including her hives, throat symptoms, and stomach pain. Her throat problems alone, with her throat-clearing and hoarse voice, were a sign that there was a problem needing epinephrine. She additionally had a history of both peanut allergy and asthma, increasing her risk of more severe reactions. So I told the nurse to go ahead and give Stacy the self-injectable epinephrine. She felt better right away and was evaluated in a local emergency room and discharged in good condition. However, I was disturbed by the way Stacy's problem had been handled by the school.

Stacy had an emergency action plan on file at the school, instructing them to give her medication if she had any potential symptoms, especially breathing problems, which was what had happened. Instead, they tried to reach her parents and then called me, allowing Stacy's allergic reaction to possibly get worse as valuable time was wasted. After this incident, I reviewed Stacy's plan with both her family and the school, making sure that they understood how important it was to give her medication immediately if she experienced any allergic symptoms, rather than trying to call her family or her physician first. Reactions can progress very rapidly at times, so it was vital for everyone to understand that epinephrine should be given right away in order to avoid any serious consequences. We also reviewed the no food sharing policy and snack supervision.

Although in this case Stacy was fine, her story points out how important it is to make sure that all communications with a school concerning a child's peanut allergy are very clear and are reviewed periodically to be certain the plan will be followed accurately.

Getting Advanced Care During an Allergic Reaction

Q: When should peanut-allergic people get medical care from an emergency room or other medical professionals?
A: There are specific times when peanut-allergic people and their families should consider going to an emergency room. They include:

• When epinephrine has been given for an allergic reaction; or

• When a significant allergic reaction has been experienced and it is not certain whether or not it is still progressing.

Q: Should you go to an emergency room or your doctor's office?
A: If you think that you're having a severe reaction, it's probably much better to go to an emergency room rather than to a doctor's office, because an emergency room is more likely to have the types of treatments that someone

might need in the event of a severe allergic reaction. Part of your emergency action plan for peanut allergy should include knowing in advance what resources are nearby.

Q: What is the best way to get there?
A: There may be some circumstances where traveling on your own is the most effective way, for example, if you could just take a few steps across the street to an emergency room. But usually the best way to get there would be in an ambulance. You should:

• Call an emergency access number like 911 and request an ambulance,

• Explain that there's an emergency and it is an allergic reaction,

• Inform them if you have given epinephrine or have epinephrine to give and that you may need additional doses, and

• Describe the symptoms.

Q: Why do you need to provide all this information?
A: The reason is that in many states, the ambulance that arrives to help you may not have epinephrine on board. So by telling the 911 operator that you may need it, they may be able to route an advanced ambulance that does have epinephrine, instead of the ambulances that do not. That would enable them to give this potentially lifesaving additional therapy, if it's needed, before getting to the hospital.

Q: Why isn't epinephrine in every ambulance?
A: Good question. We are trying to get it into every ambulance in the country, but there are some technical problems, some of them financial and some having to do with training. Emergency medical technicians (EMTs) who are basic EMTs may not have been trained in how or when to use epinephrine. You might trust them to figure it out more than you might trust someone who has no health care education, but it still does take training. And there are thousands of emergency workers who need to go through training.

In addition, the injectable devices have to be updated every year, which can be costly. Some states have gotten all these things into place, but even then, the coverage isn't 100 percent yet. So legislation is needed, and that is exactly what is happening now. But it's on a state-by-state level, and fewer than half the states have the program in place right now.

Q: What happens when the ambulance arrives?
A: Typically, the ambulance personnel will assess the situation in regard to:

• How the person with the allergic reaction is breathing, and

• How his or her circulation is functioning.

Potentially, they can give additional medication if it's available to them, or they can assist the person in giving his or her own medications.

So the primary aim of the ambulance personnel is to get the person to advanced care quickly, but they may also have the ability to give some medications en route to the emergency room, if needed.

Q: What happens in the emergency room?
A: Similar to the routine that we just reviewed for the ambulance, you would usually be triaged, meaning that the severity of your symptoms would be assessed. If it's an allergic reaction, the emergency room staff would typically bring you or your child into a treatment room right away for further evaluation. They would:

- Check your breathing, your circulation, your blood pressure, and your heart rate;

- Listen to you breathe;

- Possibly use monitor devices to see how well your body is functioning in terms of getting oxygen; and

- Monitor your blood pressure.

Q: If you're not having a severe reaction, but you have a history of prior severe reactions, will you be taken for treatment right away?
A: Not necessarily. If you come in and have no symptoms and are "stable," the emergency room staff may wait and observe you. But if you have even minor symptoms, they should take you quickly.

For instance, if you come in covered with hives and wheezing, they should get you into the emergency room and get the treatments going right away.

Q: What advice might you get when you leave the emergency room?
A: Unfortunately, recent studies show that people coming into the emergency room with allergic reactions may not get

very much advice at all on discharge. One of the main issues in regard to the emergency room visit is how long you should stay there for observation. We will discuss that next. But when you're finally discharged from the emergency room, it would be helpful to think about several things.

First, was the allergic reaction explainable? In other words, was there a known exposure to peanut, or was there an allergic reaction that could have been from anything else? This is something that you might want to discuss with the emergency room doctor while it's fresh in your mind, and also write down notes for yourself to discuss later on with your allergist. Because it's always possible that you've assumed that what happened was a reaction to peanut, when actually there may be some other allergic reaction that happened, and it would be important to think about that.

If there was some other food involved or some other exposure involved, you should be discussing that with the emergency room doctor and, later on, discussing it further with your allergist. You should talk about what those triggers might have been, so you know to avoid them until more evaluation can be done.

For example, if there was a bee sting, that would be pretty straightforward. If there was a food that you thought was safe, but that you reacted to, maybe it would turn out that it had tree nuts in it, and maybe you weren't worried about tree nuts before, but maybe you've become allergic to them. Things like that are something important to think about.

Second, if you're in the emergency room and you've used your self-injectable epinephrine, you're going to need a refill. So you're going to want to make sure that you mention it to the emergency room doctor and also *get a prescription for your refill*. You also should discuss the exact symptoms that were observed in the emergency room and what you should look out for in the hours afterwards. In many circumstances, where there's been a significant reaction, the doctor in the emergency room might prescribe antihistamines or steroids to be used for a day or two after the reaction.

Q: How long should patients remain in the emergency room after they seem to be well?
A: That is a tricky question. There is a pattern of reaction called a "biphasic," or late-phase reaction. There are studies showing that a person could have initial symptoms of an allergic reaction that may be modest in severity, and then after they've taken some medications, they may have no symptoms left, only to have symptoms recur and actually be more severe than previously an hour to several hours after those initial symptoms.

There have actually been deaths among people who were discharged from the emergency room too soon, because they seemed perfectly well; however, they had a recurrence of severe symptoms and were unable to get back to the emergency room in time for more treatment. The exact amount of time to stay in the emergency room probably depends on some of the specifics of the reaction that was experienced. But we generally advise people who have experienced a peanut-allergic reaction to *stay in the emergency room at least four hours after symptoms have resolved.* Longer waiting periods are suggested for more serious reactions.

Q: If there are problems with recovery, what else can be done in the hospital?
A: If someone's symptoms are not resolving from their peanut-allergic reaction, additional treatments are available in the hospital. For example, if there's a significant problem with blood pressure, there are medications that can be given intravenously to help the heart beat stronger and maintain normal blood pressure. If there are problems with breathing, there are machines called "respirators" to assist with that. And medications can be given to try to help open up the breathing tubes.

Doctors can also use oxygen, the medications mentioned previously, and other drugs that can help to block an allergic response. In some rare circumstances, allergic reactions could be so severe that they would need to be treated in the intensive care unit, sometimes for many days.

Case History

RUBEN

When six-year-old Ruben came to see me for a further evaluation of his peanut allergy, his family told me that he had recently had a severe reaction, and they felt they needed more information. Ruben had been diagnosed at the age of two and had experienced some mild reactions, but this was his first severe one.

The family had been on vacation and were having some ice cream at a small shop. They had asked several questions about the products to make sure Ruben got a flavor that had no peanuts in it, yet within a few minutes of eating his ice cream, Ruben had an itchy throat and began vomiting. He was given epinephrine and an antihistamine and taken to a nearby urgent care clinic.

At the clinic, Ruben's breathing, blood pressure, and oxygen were all checked, and when everything seemed fine, they sent him out. But about an hour later, Ruben became pale and was wheezing, so the family gave him another dose of epinephrine and returned to the medical facility, where he received additional treatment. He was then sent to a nearby hospital. Fortunately, with additional medication and monitoring, Ruben's symptoms improved over the next twenty-four hours, and he was well again. But the family was disturbed by the severity of his reaction, how it became better and then worse, and wanted to know if there was anything else they could do for their child.

In our discussion, I reminded them that reactions don't automatically get worse from time to time but remain unpredictable. So just because Ruben had this severe reaction, it didn't mean his next reaction would necessarily be even worse. Second, they had asked the right questions in the ice cream parlor, but they should remember that eating in this type of store can be risky, since they often use the same scoop for different types of ice cream and also scatter peanut-containing toppings on top of the ice cream, so cross-contamination with peanut can easily occur. Third, they need to remember that severe reactions can sometimes appear to resolve and then come back an hour or more later. That's why peanut-allergic people having reactions need to remain in a medical facility for observation for at least several hours. If necessary, you can remind the hospital staff about this and then sit in the waiting room for a few hours until you are certain everything is all right.

Ruben's family felt much better after our discussion, since they recognized the places where errors had been made and were resolved to be more aware of what to do in the future in order to protect their son.

18

Understanding Risks

Q: How often should someone with a peanut allergy expect to have a reaction?
A: I wish the answer could be "never again." The frequency of peanut-allergic reactions is incredibly variable, because it depends on both how careful you are and what your sensitivity is. In other words, if you're very sensitive to a small amount, you might be more likely to experience a reaction to trace amounts of peanut in various food items than you would if these small amounts don't bother you. In our studies of young children with peanut allergy, a reaction was observed on average about once every other year, ranging from mild reactions to more severe ones. But it's certainly also possible to essentially go for a lifetime without a reaction.

Q: How likely is it for reactions to be severe?
A: That is another tricky question, because it's going to depend on your sensitivity and your underlying health problems. It also depends on how you define "severe."

In terms of a fatal reaction, it is a rare event. It is much more likely for a person with a peanut allergy to die from some cause other than peanut over their lifetime. In regard to any given reaction being "severe," from the studies we've done in the general population, approximately 80 percent of peanut-allergic individuals have experienced peanut-allergic reactions that include either respiratory reactions or reactions where more than one area of the body is affected.

If you define "severe" as being treated with epinephrine, several of our studies of peanut-allergic individuals show that about 15 to 20 percent of people with a peanut allergy have used epinephrine for a reaction. However, a lot of people with more significant symptoms may not have used epinephrine, and perhaps they should have.

Q: How likely is it for someone to die from a peanut-allergic reaction?
A: An estimated 100 to 150 Americans die each year from peanut-allergic reactions. There have been a variety of different statistical calculations of the risk of dying from peanut allergy, and there is really no one way of calculating it accurately. But the risk of dying from peanut-allergic reactions is a very low one, particularly if you are educated about avoidance and prepared to treat a reaction.

Studies of fatal food-allergic reactions reveal that those at risk are those who have a known peanut allergy, underlying asthma, and did not receive epinephrine promptly during a reaction. The most troubling issue is that these risks were primarily identified among teenagers and young adults. In addition, the fatalities were likely to occur outside of the home. These observations

underscore that we need to educate our teenagers and
young adults with peanut allergy to emphasize to them
the importance of:.

• Avoidance of peanut;

• The tools they need to obtain safe meals;

• The need to have readily available emergency medications and to use them;

• The need to enlist the help of those around them, including friends, to keep them safe; and

• The need to have increased caution and instructions when
eating outside the home.

On the other hand, these observations also indicate that
ultimately, it's going to be very unusual to die from peanut
allergy, unless:

• You are not educated about peanut allergy and avoidance
issues, or

• You are denying your symptoms and delaying therapy, or

• You are almost purposely living dangerously.

In other words, because you are an educated consumer,
you are going to protect yourself in several different and
critical ways.

Living with a Peanut Allergy

In Part Four, we will discuss many of the issues of day-to-day living with a peanut allergy. When you or your child has a potentially life-threatening condition, life can be very stressful. But there are many things you can do to make sure that the environment and activities in the peanut-allergic person's life are safe, healthy, and as free from worries as possible. Once again, this depends on your knowledge of exactly what to do and your ability to follow recommendations at all times, so that even if an unexpected emergency occurs, you will be prepared, and the outcome will be a good one.

19

Some Important Issues about Living with a Peanut Allergy

Q: What general advice do you give for children or adults who are living with a peanut allergy?
A: One of the most important things I tell my patients and their families is, "I would like you or your child to have the most normal day-to-day existence possible for someone with a peanut allergy. What that usually means is that you can and should do essentially everything that everyone else does, except for eating peanut. So you should have the ability to be an active participant in life, to go to birthday parties, to go to school, and to go out to a restaurant. You just have to remember to do all these things using the knowledge that prevents you from eating peanut."

Q: Is it necessary to carry self-injectable epinephrine with you all the time?
A: The Food Allergy & Anaphylaxis Network (see resources), which is a lay organization for people with food allergies, has come up with an epigram that "accidents are

not planned." So yes, you should have your emergency medications at all times, even if you're not expecting to eat something. There are several reasons why.

Even though you might not be expecting to eat anything, you might have an unexpected opportunity to do so. And if you don't have your medication with you, you won't be able to help yourself. That's exactly the scenario where deaths have been most common. In addition, it is a good habit to always bring your medications along to reduce the chance of forgetting. So my answer is, *Have your allergy medication with you at all times, in particular the self-injectable epinephrine, even if you don't expect to be needing it.*

I also suggest that you double-check to make sure you have your medication every time you go out, because sometimes people change their clothes or handbags and later discover they forgot to take along their medication. It is a good habit to select convenient ways to carry the medications and written instructions, in order to reduce the risk of forgetting. For example, using a fanny pack that is always worn or a knapsack or purse that is always taken along could reduce the chance of forgetting the medications. And I also suggest having jewelry that identifies your allergy.

Q: Why is it necessary to have medical-identification jewelry?
A: The use of medical alert jewelry—a bracelet or necklace that says you are allergic to peanut (see resources)—is suggested. In this way, if a reaction occurs and the allergic person is unable to explain his or her allergy (for example, if he or she cannot speak or is unconscious), the identification bracelet will alert a rescuer that this is a person with

an allergy, so they can consider the possibility of an allergic reaction in dealing with the medical emergency.

For most people, just having a diagnosis of peanut allergy warrants wearing medical-identification jewelry. There may be some younger children who are always surrounded by people who really know what their medical history issues are and know to protect them, so with that age group you might consider not needing identification jewelry as much. But especially as children get older and spend more time with friends in places where people who know them are not necessarily available, they would certainly benefit from wearing this identification jewelry. And starting with the jewelry at a younger age may promote good habits for later years.

Q: How vigilant does someone have to be regarding avoidance of peanut?
A: The simple answer here is to be very vigilant. I always advise people to be very vigilant about whatever they're eating, to ask questions and to give explanations to people who are providing food to them, and to always consider that any food they are getting could potentially have peanut in it, so having emergency medical treatment available all the time is part of vigilance. Therefore, those with peanut allergy should always make sure they are doing whatever is necessary in order to be certain their food is safe. Never forget that even a small amount of ingested peanut can trigger a reaction, possibly a severe one, and you never want to leave that as an open possibility.

Having said all of that, there could also be an overinterpretation of vigilance; that is, avoiding circumstances that pose little risk, to the point that day-to-day activities become hampered and quality of life is suffering unnecessarily. Hopefully, the pointers in this book and the advice from your physician will prevent this from occurring.

Lastly, "vigilance" should include maintaining an emergency action plan.

Q: What is an "emergency action plan"?
A: An "emergency action plan" is a term that really encompasses several things. One is that it means that emergency medications are available and that the people who may be using them for themselves or for others know how to use them and when to use them and also how to activate professional assistance. For example, they know to call 911 and how to describe the situation to a 911 operator.

In addition, an emergency action plan often includes something available in writing. So when we talk about what to do for children in school settings or in camp settings a little farther on in this book, you will see that a *written emergency plan* becomes a key part of your overall general care plan.

An emergency plan also extends a general care plan for peanut allergy. The general plan includes information about the allergy for those who have it or for those who are caring for someone who has it. That means understanding what the symptoms are and understanding what the avoidance issues are, in order to keep the peanut allergic person safe.

20

The Amount That Causes a Reaction

Q: Is it true that a trace amount of peanut can cause a reaction?
A: In short, yes. There are several studies that have investigated the amount of ingested peanut that may cause a reaction. The studies show a range of results. There are studies showing that very minuscule amounts of peanut can cause some symptoms for a minority of very sensitive people. However, in most of the studies where individuals are purposely fed peanut to see if they will react, the amount that causes objective symptoms—meaning more than just an itchy mouth or a "sensation," for example—is typically in the range of 3 to 200 milligrams, which essentially is a small but typically visible amount of peanut (from about one-fiftieth to one-half of a peanut kernel). In one large study of adults who had significant peanut allergy and were purposely fed peanut, reactions requiring treatment were elicited when, on average, about one-half of a peanut kernel was ingested.

Q: Is there a relationship between the amount of peanut eaten and the severity of the reaction?
A: There have been no studies that have specifically addressed the question of whether the amount you eat is related to the severity of a reaction, but most physicians would assume that there is. In other words, the more that you've ingested, the more likely it is that a reaction would be severe. And that would mean conversely that there are people who ingest trace or small or sometimes even modest amounts of peanut and might have no symptoms at all.

Q: Is there a way to predict the amount of peanut that would cause a reaction for any individual person?
A: Unfortunately, there is currently no way to predict this. In the studies that have been conducted so far, a reaction to a particular amount of exposure has not related perfectly to your blood level of peanut IgE antibody or to the test size of your peanut allergy skin test. It's surprising that it's not the case, because you would imagine that the higher your test is, the smaller an amount that would trigger a reaction, or that there would be more of a relationship for a severe reaction. But it just doesn't turn out that way, and so far, we don't know why.

There are some people who actually tolerate fairly large amounts of peanut with never more than an itchy mouth. We believe these individuals are allergic to a specific protein in peanut that is essentially less potent than other proteins in peanut, but there are currently no tests to accurately identify such individuals.

21

Skin and Inhalation Exposures

Q: Can someone have a reaction from just touching or smelling peanut?
A: The answer is "yes and no." Or more accurately, "it depends."

If you have skin contact with peanut, the most common symptom to expect is an allergic reaction that happens exactly at the point of contact. This is essentially the same situation that we see when we do an allergy skin test to peanut.

During an allergy skin prick/scratch test to peanut, we put an extract (a diluted amount of peanut) on the skin and scratch the skin in order to get the protein to seep in. We then watch the area swell, which is similar to a mosquito-bite reaction if someone is potentially allergic. But we do not expect that person to have a reaction anywhere else on the body. Similarly, if you are allergic and have peanut rubbed on your skin, you might expect some redness in the place where it touches, but it would be very unusual for a reaction to occur anywhere else on the body.

In regard to smelling peanut, that is also a situation that depends on the circumstances, partly because peanut butter is an oily substance, and peanut protein does not come off of peanut butter very well at all.

We did a study that was funded through the Food Allergy Initiative, a lay organization that raises funds for research in food allergy and is also involved in education and legislation for the benefit of food-allergic individuals (see resources), to investigate casual contact with peanut butter. We enrolled thirty highly peanut-allergic children who sniffed peanut butter that was disguised, so that they couldn't detect the peanut smell. Their noses were one foot away from peanut butter for ten minutes while they were sniffing, and no one had a reaction at all. Other investigators have tried to measure peanut protein in the air very close to peanut butter and were unable to find any.

The situation might be different if you were dealing with peanut flour, which is a powdery substance. If you were cooking with peanut flour, it presumably could become airborne much more readily and might cause some problems with inhalation.

Q: What if you touch peanut? For example, if there is some peanut on a table and a child touches her elbow with it?
A: That is a potentially common scenario in a school setting. Perhaps a child has left a smear of peanut butter on a table, and another child comes and touches it. If it has just touched the skin, we would expect a reaction only on the skin at the point of contact, and possibly no reaction at all.

We did a study where we took thirty highly peanut-allergic children and rubbed a pea-sized amount of peanut butter on their skin, left it there for a minute, and then wiped it away. Only about a third of the children developed any reaction, and for them, all that happened was a red blotch or hive in that area. The majority had no response at all. Again, this is similar to a skin test. And in fact, the reason two-thirds of the children did not have a response may be that we put the peanut butter on intact skin without scratching the surface of the skin. For a diagnostic allergy skin test, we scratch the skin to see a response.

So there are some nuances here. One is that if a person has eczema, which is an itchy skin rash where the skin is sometimes broken open, you might expect more of a reaction if peanut butter is rubbed on a spot like that.

The other nuance is contact with the eyes. The eye is almost like a large open area, where direct exposure to a small amount of what you're allergic to can cause a lot of symptoms. Think about people with pollen allergies who go outside on a day with high pollen counts. They get red, itchy, and swollen eyes from exposure to nearly invisible amounts of pollen flying into their eyes. So if you're peanut-allergic and you touch peanut on your finger and then rub it into your eye, you might expect a tremendous amount of eyelid swelling; sometimes the eyes may even swell shut. That can look quite dramatic, although again, it would be very unlikely to progress beyond the eye.

Q: How can I clean peanut off hands, dishes, or tables sufficiently to prevent a problem?
A: There was actually a study looking at the efficacy of a variety of types of cleaning methods for tables and hands. What it really boils down to is that using soap with running water is the best way to get peanut sufficiently off your

hands. When individuals actually smeared peanut butter on their hands, washed afterwards with soap and water until they didn't see any left, and then did assays of their hands—which is a scientific method of trying to detect peanut on the skin—they found no peanut. Commercial wet wipes were also effective.

Similarly, in the study they washed tables with a variety of different materials and found that just washing with water and a wipe until the table was clean left the table with no detectable peanut, even though peanut butter had been on the table previously. Several other cleansers also worked, including Formula 409, Target cleaner with bleach, and Lysol wipes.

Q: Were there any cleaning methods that did not work well?
A: For hand cleaning, if they used water with no soap, a tiny bit of peanut was detected on some hands. The hand-cleaning method that didn't work well at all was waterless antibacterial soap, which you sometimes come across in zoos and similar places where running water is not readily available. With these waterless cleaners, you don't wash your hands, you just rub an antibacterial material on your hands. It turns out that these agents do not help to rid the hands of peanut residue, which is not a surprise, because the peanut can never actually get off your fingers completely if there's no running water.

When tables were cleaned, as mentioned above, plain water and wiping did fine, with no detectable residue. Several cleansers were also successful, but dishwashing liquid left detectable residue on some tables, possibly because of having left a thin film that was not wiped off.

Q: What about dishwashing liquid in dishwashers?
A: The researchers did not study that issue, but the circumstances of a dishwasher are different from wiping a tabletop with dishwashing liquid. In a dishwasher, dishes and utensils are rinsed, soaped, and rinsed again. While there are no studies, it seems that such a routine is closer to the hand-washing routine and likely to efficiently remove peanut (assuming, of course, that the dishes were prerinsed and not left with large amounts of peanut butter on them prior to washing).

Q: What if you wipe off your hands with a dry tissue or paper towel afterward?
A: That's probably not good enough, because you're still not getting the dilution effect of running water or the effect of a wet wipe that also worked in the study.

Q: When you're cleaning up, if you can't see any peanut, do you still need to worry?
A: In regard to cleaning things like dishes, utensils, and tabletops, if you can't see any peanut, and you have cleaned in a way described above, you probably don't need to worry about it anymore.

There was a study where the investigators went through six preschools and schools in which there was no special cleaning beforehand, but one school was "peanut-free," and they tested the tables and food preparation areas, desks, and water fountains by wiping them and then they ran an assay to detect whether there was peanut on those items. None of thirty-six eating areas and none of twenty-two desks had detectable peanut protein. One of thirteen water fountains had detectable peanut, but the amount was very low and was an amount that virtually no one would ever have reacted to, even if they licked the whole area. So the bottom line appears to be this: If you can't see any peanut on an item not meant to be licked, it is most likely safe. If you cannot see peanut on an item used for eating that has been cleaned in a way described previously, it is probably safe.

Q: Are some forms of peanut more dangerous than others?
A: There are two issues in this question. The first issue regards how different forms of peanut may behave in regard to exposure. Peanut butter, being an oily substance where the peanut protein does not come off of it, probably poses less of an issue than, for example, peanut flour, which might be used in cooking and can get airborne. Also, roasted peanuts in bags can theoretically pose a problem, because when you pop open the bag, you might get peanut dust into the air, which could cause some symptoms. Or if you're cracking open peanuts in their shells, you might also get some peanut dust into the air.

Interestingly, a recently published study attempted to detect peanut protein in the air next to peanut butter, shelled peanuts, and unshelled peanuts, and could not detect any. I tried this same experiment and also could not detect peanut. While it may be that the laboratory tests were not sensitive enough to detect very minute amounts, there certainly does not seem to be any large amounts of exposure in these settings.

The second issue regards whether airborne peanut protein would be intrinsically more potent than, for example, airborne proteins from cat, pollen, or other typically airborne allergens. I don't know of any scientific evidence that indicates that inhaling a little bit of peanut protein is more of an issue than, for example, if someone with an allergy to cats inhales a bit of cat protein if a cat is around or if a person with hay fever to pollens inhales pollen in the pollen season.

The symptoms I might expect in these circumstances, be it airborne peanut protein, cat dander, or pollen, might be itchy eyes, a runny nose, or nasal congestion. And if someone has asthma and an allergy to these items and they have inhaled any of them, it might possibly trigger an asthma reaction. But I would not normally expect small exposures to cause a drop in blood pressure, for example.

Q: What if an allergic person smells peanut, for instance on an airplane?
A: An airplane is an unusual situation, because you may have 200 people opening packets of peanuts at the same time. They are powdery peanuts and with a small air space, it is quite possible that peanut protein could become airborne.

In fact, there was a study looking at the protein from peanut that collected in airplane air filters left in place over months of flight, and peanut protein was readily detectable in those filters. So some of the protein seems to get into the air and circulate. The issue is, would this cause a significant problem for a child or adult with a peanut allergy? And the answer to that is still a bit unclear.

Q: Have any studies been done on this issue?
A: Yes. We did a study using our registry of people with peanut and/or tree nut allergies that we maintain in con-

junction with The Food Allergy & Anaphylaxis Network.
At the time of the study, there were 3,704 people in the
registry, in which people described their symptoms from
peanut allergy in a variety of settings, and of these, 35 described reactions they had experienced on or associated
with an airplane. We contacted these individuals to discuss
what happened to them on the airplane.

For fourteen people, the reason for the reaction was that
they actually ate peanut on the airplane; seven were touching peanut; and fourteen attributed a reaction to inhalation
of peanut. All of the skin contact reactions were mild and
only affected the skin. Among those who ate peanut, three
had severe symptoms. Most of the ingestion reactions were
among very young children, some who ate peanut for the
first time and some who apparently found peanut on a seat.
For the fourteen who attributed reactions to inhalation,
there were a variety of specific circumstances. Ten people
described only minimal or mild symptoms, two described
moderate symptoms, and two described severe symptoms.
Of the two people with more severe symptoms, they were
not certain the reaction had to do with peanut (one had
symptoms before peanut was served, one forty minutes after peanut had been served.)

**Q: What conclusions about air travel can be drawn from this
study?**
A: In general, putting together the results from several
studies and also a few individual reports, it seems that air
exposure to peanut on commercial flights is an issue for
some but certainly not the vast majority of peanut-allergic
individuals, and there is a small possibility for more serious symptoms. However, the concern for ingestion re-

actions in young peanut-allergic children is a significant issue.

What I generally recommend for my patients who are going on an airplane is that they be extremely careful about what is around their young child with peanut allergy. You have to:

• Make sure that your child doesn't pick up a peanut that was left between the seats or on the floor, and eat it;

• Look at or wipe off the trays that come down in front of the seats to make sure there isn't any food left over on them; and

• Look in the pockets in front of the seats to make sure that someone hasn't left some food that your child might grab.

In regard to eating on the airplane, it's always safest to *bring your own food*, if you can. Or at least discuss with the airline in advance how they may be able to provide you with a safe meal. However, you may not always find that you feel completely safe about the food available on airplanes, so it may just be safer and less stressful to have your own food with you.

Q: Do airlines ever have peanut-free flights?
A: In recent years, some of the airlines have been providing peanut-free snacks, particularly if you call ahead and request them. But the exact rules about peanuts and flying are still not completely worked out. The Food Allergy & Anaphylaxis Network has specific peanut-related information on some of the airlines, which changes frequently and should be checked prior to your flight. Some airlines will

clear three rows ahead and behind the person with a peanut allergy so that the individuals in those rows are not opening up packs of peanuts close to the allergic person. I also tell families that if they fly in the morning, it's less likely that peanuts will be served. The airlines do not want to use the term "peanut-free flight" because, while they may agree not to serve peanuts on a given flight, they cannot control what their passengers may bring on board, which may include peanuts.

There have not been studies regarding peanut proteins emanating from peanut while they are being roasted or heated. Until such studies are done, I would be concerned about flights that actually roast or heat peanut, which is apparently sometimes done in First Class. (See chapter 28 for more information on air travel.)

Q: In general, what do you advise your patients regarding casual exposure to peanut?
A: Because an ingestion exposure can follow some of the casual exposures, it's always important to keep in mind that, especially for younger children who are prone to putting fingers or toys in their mouths, you want to try to reduce any exposure to peanut. So it would not alarm me if people with a peanut allergy touched peanut on their fingers and then washed their hands, but it would alarm me if I saw a peanut-allergic two-year-old touching peanut and then having it on the fingers, because a young child is very likely to put fingers in the mouth, and that could easily cause a problem. Young children could also easily touch peanut and then rub their eyes, which can cause dramatic swelling there.

For older individuals, the main potentially severe type of casual contact is from kissing.

Q: So kissing could be a problem for peanut-allergic people?
A: Yes, but the impact of the exposure can vary. If someone has been eating peanut and is going to kiss a person
with peanut allergy, there can be a transfer of peanut protein in the kiss. So what I typically tell families is that if
Grandma is eating peanut butter and then kisses Johnny on
the cheek, his cheek might get red where she kissed it, but
I still would not expect Johnny to get sick anywhere else in
his body, as we previously discussed. But if Grandma gave
Johnny a mouth-to-mouth "wet" kiss, there could be a
problem, because peanut protein could be transferred into
Johnny's mouth and ingested.

Intimate kissing is a major concern for older individuals
if one partner has been eating peanut. In that situation,
saliva with peanut protein could cause a severe, anaphylactic reaction because the situation is similar to ingestion of
peanut. Therefore, kissing is an important issue for
teenagers and older age groups who have peanut allergy,
because they need to discuss their allergies with their dates
or partners to be certain that they have not been eating
peanut or peanut butter prior to any intimate kissing. (See
chapter 22 for more information about kissing and intimate
contact.)

**Q: Is there any test to find out if someone is extremely sensi-
tive to peanut, such that casual exposure by smell or touch is
more dangerous?**
A: There are no simple allergy laboratory tests for severity.
While several of the studies I have discussed indicate that
severe reactions from casual exposure to peanut butter are
not a typical concern for most people with peanut allergy,
there are reports of single individuals who seem to have

experienced severe reactions from minimal exposure by touch or smell.

It is hard to scientifically verify such reports. In other words, it is often difficult to determine whether or not some peanut was eaten or if there was another cause of the reaction. I have described our study of thirty children with severe peanut allergy who did not have a significant reaction to skin contact or any reaction to the smell of peanut butter. It is not possible to generalize from that study that absolutely no peanut-allergic person is at risk from similar exposures, and we did not do tests on other forms of peanut (such as peanut flour), nor did we coat large areas of skin with peanut butter.

However, I view the study as encouraging for most situations and for most people with peanut allergy. I therefore emphasize that ingestion of peanut, including tiny amounts, is the major concern, including the concern that a casual exposure can lead to ingestion, particularly in young children who are more likely to lick objects and fingers.

Q: What if there is a remaining concern that touching or smelling peanut may cause a severe reaction?
A: There are families or individuals who are very concerned about the types of casual exposures that we have discussed here. To specifically address this issue of casual exposure for you or your child with peanut allergy, I would suggest a discussion with your allergist. Some allergists may determine that a "re-creation" of the study I performed in the form of a challenge test is right for you.

We specifically did these studies to try to see whether this type of contact causes problems, and we did not find it to be a problem. But if any patients or their families have difficulty with this issue, it would be possible to re-create what we did in the study and see if any reactions beyond the skin occur.

We conducted our study of casual contact to peanut so that the children being tested did not know whether they were actually being touched with peanut or something that was not peanut (that is, a placebo). They also did not know whether they were sniffing peanut butter or were sniffing another substance that was masked to smell the same (we used tuna, soy, and mint.) We "masked" the test materials because people are often nervous and may respond in ways that mimic an allergy, even if no reaction is happening. In fact, there was one child who had some symptoms during the time she was sniffing the test material—she felt that her throat was itchy—but it turned out that her reaction was actually to the placebo that did not have any peanut butter in it, so it was more of a nervous reaction.

Case History

JENNIFER

Diagnosed at the age of two with peanut allergy, Jennifer was a seven-year-old who had been homeschooled, primarily because her family was afraid that she could be exposed to peanut at school. Jennifer's blood test for peanut allergy was at the top of the scale, so her parents felt she was at risk for a severe reaction, though she had just a mild reaction when she was two years old and another mild one at the age of three. She came to me because her parents had recently been discussing the need for homeschooling; her father felt she should be in school with the other children, and her mother felt it was unsafe.

In our discussion, Jennifer's mother said she was especially worried that her daughter might touch or smell peanut at school and would have a bad reaction. The parents explained that when Jennifer was three years old, her grandmother had wiped her face with a dishrag that had some peanut butter on it, and Jennifer's entire face became swollen, with her eyes swollen shut, so the family was very worried about the severity of her allergy.

I retested Jennifer, and she still had very high IgE antibody levels to peanut (over 100 kIU/L). I explained to her family that even though Jennifer had a very high test score, that did not necessarily mean that her reactions would be severe every time she was exposed to a small amount of peanut by casual exposure. I also told them that most peanut-allergic people do not have significant reactions from casual contact with peanut. I also pointed out that although homeschooling can be effective, if it was being undertaken only because of the peanut allergy, they may want to reconsider whether or not it was a necessary undertaking. Indeed, Jennifer wanted to go to school with the children she knew from town and promised her family she would only eat foods that were safe.

Because the family was so worried that touching or smelling peanut could trigger a severe reaction, I did a food challenge with Jennifer, where we touched her with peanut butter and also had her smell it. In both cases, nothing happened, which was very reassuring to the family. As a result of this test and our discussion, Jennifer's mother decided to let her go to school in the fall and began working on the emergency action and care plans that would be set up to insure that Jennifer would not be exposed to peanut, and if she was, the school would know exactly how to handle it.

22.

Special Issues in Avoidance

Q: What are some of the major trouble areas for people living with peanut allergy?

A: Most of the pitfalls experienced by individuals living with peanut allergy typically occur when they are eating outside of their homes, particularly in restaurants, friends' homes, or other places where food is being prepared outside of their immediate supervision and control. But there are a few more unusual exposure situations that I am sometimes asked about that can be a problem, and these include exposure from:

• Saliva,

• Intimate contact,

• Blood transfusions, and

• Breast-feeding.

Q: By "saliva," you mean kissing is the issue?
A: Not just kissing! Sometimes people share drinking cups, straws, utensils, and the like. For example, this issue extends to a warm day when a group of children might be tempted to share a drink from the same can or sharing cups and the like within a family. If a person ate peanut and was using a straw and then a peanut-allergic person used the same straw, there could be a transfer of some peanut protein that could be ingested. A well-meaning taste could be dangerous. This issue should be reviewed with the peanut-allergic individual and with those who supervise peanut-allergic children.

Q: What do peanut-allergic people need to know about kissing and dating?
A: As we previously mentioned, one potential problem is intimate kissing between someone who has ingested peanut and someone who's allergic. The reason is that an exchange of saliva could contain peanut and cause an actual allergic reaction. This could be a potentially serious issue, especially with teenagers who may be reluctant to discuss their allergies. So those with peanut allergies who are involved in close relationships must remember to discuss their allergies with their partners and make sure that the partner has not ingested peanut or peanut-containing products near the time that they are engaged in intimate kissing.

Unfortunately, at this time we do not have results of studies on the residual amounts of peanut in saliva after peanut or peanut-containing products have been eaten at various times after eating food or after brushing teeth or rinsing the mouth. Until such data are available, I suggest that intimate kissing should not follow ingestion of peanut foods for at least an hour or more, according to what was eaten and following very thorough brushing and rinsing by the person who has eaten peanut.

Q: Can peanut protein get into other bodily fluids in regard to intimate contact?
A: It is clear that peanut protein gets into the bloodstream, so there could be a theoretical concern of an allergic reaction to semen. In fact, there are women who are allergic to semen, but these allergies have been identified as a response to actual semen proteins, not to peanut proteins in semen. There was one report, not given in any detail, of a possible reaction to walnut protein in semen, but saliva transfer could have been the trigger. At this time, there are no reports of an allergic reaction to semen due to transfer of peanut protein.

Q: If someone with peanut allergy needs a blood transfusion and the blood donor has consumed peanuts, could that present a problem?
A: When you ingest peanut, a small amount of the protein gets into your bloodstream. Therefore, if you give a donation of your blood, there may be a small amount of the peanut protein you've ingested in the blood itself.

However, calculations have been done in regard to the amount of protein that would be in the bloodstream and the amount that would end up in a transfusion. The blood cells are concentrated, so that the liquid part of the blood donation, where the peanut protein would reside, is largely removed. As a result, the amount that would be residual in any given unit of blood, even for someone who has ingested a normal serving of peanuts, would be extremely low and highly unlikely to trigger a reaction. There have been no reports of an allergic reaction from this in the scientific literature. Overall, there seems to be little to support a concern. However, if you were getting so-called "donor-directed" blood for an elective operation, the donors might as well be asked to avoid peanut before their donation to eliminate any remaining concern. In regard to how long to avoid it, this has not been studied, but it seems that twelve to twenty-four hours would suffice.

There are several reports of peanut allergy being transferred from an organ donor or bone marrow donor who has peanut allergy to a transplant recipient who does not have a peanut allergy. This would not be an issue for blood transfusions because cells capable of transferring an allergy are not viable in normal circumstances of blood donation.

Q: If a mother is breast-feeding and knows that her child has a peanut allergy, and she accidentally ate peanut, could that be a problem?
A: The peanut protein that a mother ingests can be transferred into her breast milk. There was a study looking at this question involving twenty-three women who were purposely eating peanut for the study, and eleven, or half of them, did pass the peanut protein into their breast milk.

The study procedure had the mothers express breast milk every hour, and then the breast milk was checked for peanut proteins. It turns out that while half of them did not transfer any peanut protein into their breast milk, the half that did had a peak in the amount they expressed at one hour after they ate peanut. By four hours after they ate peanut, all but two did not have any more detectable peanut protein in their breast milk. Two of the participants did have peanut detectable in their breast milk beyond four hours, and one of them had it for up to eight hours. The study didn't look at that person beyond eight hours, so it could have theoretically remained even longer.

The conclusion is that, ultimately, if you ingest peanut while breast-feeding, there is a chance that there could be peanut protein in your breast milk. So if you know that your infant is allergic, you may want to express and discard your milk for at least six or eight hours before trying to give it to your baby.

23.

Food Shopping

Q: **What advice do you give those who are peanut-allergic in regard to food shopping?**
A: My general advice is to *read every label very carefully* in regard to the possibility that there's going to be peanut in that food. My specific instructions may include particular problems that come up in special settings, which will be covered in the questions that follow.

Q: **Where in the process of food shopping can mistakes happen?**
A: It would be nice if we could pick up a product, read the label, and know off the bat whether it has peanut. Unfortunately, it is not that simple for several reasons. First, label reading can be tricky; and second, the label may be inaccurate. One important issue is the way that labels are worded. If you look at the ingredients list on a product, you might not see anything about peanuts, but then there may be a warning elsewhere on the label that says, "May Contain

Peanuts." Sometimes this warning is very close to the ingredients list, but sometimes it isn't. So if you don't look all around the label, you may miss it. Of course, sometimes it's written in very prominent letters that you can't miss, but not always.

Another tricky aspect about label reading can be summed up by my suggestion to check the label every time, even if you have bought the product before. These labels can change if manufacturing changes. Believe it or not, sometimes different-size packages of the same product may have slightly different ingredients.

The second issue is one of accuracy. In particular, smaller companies or individual stores may have incomplete or inaccurate labeling or may not consider issues of cross-contact in their processing. For example, there may be ingredients in a bakery store product that are not included on the label. The burden for the consumer right now is unfortunate. You should have higher suspicions about smaller stores and products, such as baked goods or nutty items, that are more likely to be made with or around peanuts.

A good example of this is cashew butter. You might purchase cashew butter because you don't have a nut allergy but only have a peanut allergy. But if they make the cashew butter right in the store and also use the same grinder to make fresh peanut butter, there's a good chance that you would have cross-contact, even though there might be no warning on the label.

Another problem is unlabeled open-barrel items in some supermarkets. You may be scooping discount chocolate cereal from a barrel, but the food could have been contaminated by a previous shopper with peanut cereal from a different barrel. Lastly, you probably cannot trust the labels of products that are made in foreign countries with different or no labeling requirements. And watch out for products where an English label is pasted over a foreign-language label.

Q: In other words, reading a label may not be sufficient?
A: In most cases, I would say that label reading is good enough. But there are some products that you may want to be particularly careful with, in particular, some confectionary products, especially those from small manufacturers. For example, the following products might contain peanut that does not appear on the label, either as an ingredient or in a warning:

• Bakery products

• Ice cream products

• Dessert products

• Candies that have peanut-containing versions/types

So, while label reading may be good enough most of the time, if you really want to be sure, you may have to do more investigation if these products are from small companies.

Q: Do you have to call the company?
A: Many times, especially for the riskier types of products, the answer is "yes." Companies have become more allergy-aware, but some smaller ones may warrant a call.

The FDA did a study of a variety of manufacturing facilities where confectionary products were made. They looked at labels and assayed the foods, which means they did a scientific test on the foods to determine if there was peanut in them. In the study, the researchers looked at peanut and also egg and milk. They found that 25 percent of the time there were mistakes in the labeling, with ingredients undeclared. So however you look at it, mistakes are being made by these confectionary companies. For that reason alone, those who are peanut-allergic should call these types of companies before using their products. The companies should at least be able to tell you if they make peanut-containing products, so you can determine if there may be some risk of cross-contamination with peanut in their other products.

In addition, many companies may use ambiguous terminology on their labels. For example, they may say "natural flavoring," and you wouldn't know for certain whether or not that was peanut—and it could be. You may be particularly suspicious if the product you want to use is the type of product where peanut may be a possible ingredient. Therefore, you would need to call the company to find out. (See appendix II for the terms regarding peanut that are definitely or sometimes indicative of a peanut ingredient.)

There are some companies specializing in peanut-free and nut-free confectionary and bakery products, which would reduce some of the burden on the consumer until labeling laws and manufacturing processes improve.

Q: What should you say when calling the food company?
A: I suggest you explain to the company that you or your child has a peanut allergy and you are not asking questions in order to find out about any secret ingredients in their products but simply to find out if their product will be safe for you. Explain that you want to know if there is any peanut protein or peanut products in the product you want

to use, regardless of whether peanut is a main ingredient; or if the product is made on equipment that makes peanut-containing foods.

In that context, the company should not feel threatened that you're trying to find out what their ingredients might be, and they should understand that your interest in their product's ingredients is solely for health reasons, that is, to be certain that it doesn't contain what you or your child is allergic to.

Many food companies have 800 numbers listed on their labels or sometimes on their Web sites, so a lot of these food companies are now making it easier for their customers to contact them.

Q: Are there any other specific food ingredients that should concern allergic customers?
A: There are some flavoring agents that may be used in dressings or barbecue sauces that could also contain peanut.

Q: How do you interpret labels that say "May Contain Peanut"?
A: There are no specific rules instructing a company exactly how to word the notice that their product may contain peanut, nor have there been guidelines as to when such terms should or should not be used. If peanut is a specific ingredient in the product, it should certainly be listed as one of the ingredients. But the issue here is, for example, that equipment used to process peanuts may also be used to make the product that you're buying, even though peanut is not intended as an ingredient. So by using the same equip-

ment, there may possibly be some carryover of peanut protein into your product that was not meant to have peanut.

Q: What can peanut-allergic people do about this kind of situation?
A: If the company indicates that the product may contain peanut by carrying the warning label "May Contain Peanut," it's always safest to assume that the specific product has peanut in it and should be avoided.

Q: Is the phrase "May Contain Peanut" the same as "Made in a Factory Where Peanut Is Processed" or other similar terms seen on product labels?
A: Because there are no specific rules or guidelines for the terms that the companies must use, you will see a variety of terms used, including these and many others. You may be tempted to assume that a phrase such as "Made in a Facility with Peanuts" is less risky than "Made on Equipment with Peanuts," but there are no guidelines associated with these phrases and no way to assess comparative risk. Some labels say "May Contain Nuts," and I would not know if they consider peanut, a legume, to be included in their use of the term "nuts." So ultimately, there is no special meaning to most of these terms. They should all be taken as warnings that peanut may be in the product and therefore should be avoided by all those who have peanut allergies.

Q: If a peanut-allergic person has been eating a product for a while without problems and then realizes it is labeled "May Contain Peanut," should they stop eating it?

A: Many people ask me this question during office visits, because once a diagnosis of peanut allergy is made and I explain avoidance to them, many families realize that they or their children have already been eating products that are labeled this way and have never had a problem.

My general answer is that I don't work for that company, and so there is no way I can know what the risk is for any given box or container of the product that is being eaten. These labels certainly are not stating that any particular box has peanut inside, but rather that there is some level of risk. If the company has decided to put a peanut warning on the label, that indicates to me that there is some finite risk. So to be safest, my recommendation to my patients is to avoid these foods. I think we have to take these labels at face value and consider that there really is a risk.

On the other hand, I understand the frustration and why some families may elect to continue to eat products they tolerated so many times without a problem. I just cannot condone this practice at this time.

Q: What about many products that have peanut oil?
A: Peanut oil is a fatty derivative of peanut. Depending on how the oil is separated from the protein of crude peanut, it may contain either virtually no peanut protein or a large amount of peanut protein. Highly processed peanut oil typically contains almost no peanut protein, and in some studies, individuals with significant peanut allergy ingested this oil with absolutely no symptoms. On the other hand, peanut oil that is derived by squeezing or extruding peanut oil from peanuts carries with it a significant amount of protein and would certainly cause a reaction for people who are allergic.

The main problem here is that you may not know from a label that says "Peanut Oil" whether it's the processed kind or the crude kind. And particularly in many of the more "gourmet" types of products, such as some cookies or potato chips, it's likely that they would use the more flavorful crude peanut oil, which can lead to problems.

Even though some types of peanut oil are likely safe, I generally recommend that my patients *avoid peanut oil* in any products, because you don't know in any given product whether it's the crude type or not.

You can also purchase highly processed peanut oil from any supermarket. According to some studies, this type of peanut oil has very little to no peanut protein, and as mentioned before, there are studies showing people with peanut allergy tolerating this type of oil. There are also some studies showing that some of these processed oils can cause a reaction in some people with peanut allergy, so the area is a bit controversial. Therefore, the issue here is one of degree of restriction, in that there may be a small amount of lot-to-lot variability with these products, and you may, at least theoretically, come across a refined peanut oil that has enough protein to actually trigger a reaction.

I have met some allergists who restrict refined peanut oil and others who do not. I fall on the side of restriction at this point in time for the specific issues that:

• You do not always know what type of peanut oil is in your store-purchased food or restaurant product; and

• It seems simple enough to select an oil other than peanut oil to cook with in order to avoid theoretical risks, pending more studies.

Q: Is it even necessary to use peanut oil to begin with?
A: Oils of this type have certain characteristics, including their individual heating points, and flavors, and sometimes peanut oil is simply the preferred oil for certain dishes. Peanut oil actually ends up in lots of products that would otherwise be safe to eat, but again, you don't know which is which in regard to refined or crude/extruded peanut oil. As a result, I think it's too much trouble to try to figure out which products are safe, so I just advise people to avoid all products with peanut oil as an ingredient.

Q: Do you have any advice in regard to keeping "unsafe" foods in your food storage areas away from peanut-allergic people?
A: In many households, the nonallergic people living there may decide to have peanut products or peanut-containing products in their homes, but those who have peanut allergies are obviously not going to eat them.

One way of trying to keep mistakes from happening is to label the unsafe products, and/or the safe products in a way that makes them easily identifiable. For example, some families will buy red tape and put it on all the products containing peanut, so everyone knows not to grab them when preparing food for the peanut-allergic person. Sometimes families will use a strip of green tape to indicate non–peanut-containing products that the person with peanut allergy can safely eat, though that usually takes a lot more effort.

Other families put aside a specific shelf in the refrigerator or cupboard where products that are not safe for the allergic person are kept. But using colored tape is probably better, since food products can accidentally be moved around from shelf to shelf, making mistakes more likely.

Q: Are there families who simply do not purchase or keep any products that have peanut as an ingredient or possible ingredient?
A: Yes, there are families who completely exclude any products that may contain peanut from their homes because they feel safer doing that.

Q: What are the implications of the new labeling laws?
A: Many of the problems that have been discussed in this section will hopefully become much less problematic as the new labeling laws are phased in, which is planned for January 2006. These new labeling laws, the Food Allergen Labeling and Consumer Protection Act, require companies to use more obvious labeling of peanut products and other food allergens. But it's important to realize that there may be a lag in terms of actual compliance with the new laws. So families are still going to have to be very wary of the labels they read, even as these laws come into effect.

Q: Is it easy to read labels accurately, or do people make mistakes?
A: We actually did a study of parents who were avoiding peanut, asking them to look at a booklet of labels. Some of those labels included terms indicating they had or may have contained peanut.

It turned out that half of the families made mistakes, where they misread labels. And the biggest mistake was made because on some of the labels, it says "May Contain Peanuts," or "Facilities with Peanuts," but those words were not right next to the ingredients label, so they didn't see them because they didn't really look around the whole label.

Therefore, my advice is that when you are reading a product label and checking for the possible presence of peanut, don't just look at the ingredients list. Be sure that you *look everywhere on the label* to see if any of the terms we have mentioned, such as "May Contain Peanut" are on the label.

24.

Going to School

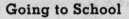

Q: Is it safe for a child with peanut allergy to attend school?
A: In general, the answer is definitely "yes," when proper preparations are made. There may be some circumstances, usually regarding some child care settings or preschools for very young children, where provisions are sometimes not adequate enough for comfort. But in most cases, a safe environment can be achieved. And certainly by the time children are in kindergarten and grade school, I would expect that a safe environment could be universally achieved, so that all children with peanut allergies can safely attend school.

Q: Why would child care centers and preschools have a problem creating a safe environment for peanut-allergic children?
A: With child care or preschool, one is required to supervise very young children who may be toddling around, cannot place any limit on themselves in regard to food sharing, and are at an oral stage where transfer of food pro-

teins by toys and furniture is an issue. While certainly not impossible, this is a particularly riskier situation that requires careful consideration in avoiding exposure to peanut. Families have to determine the "lay of the land" in regard to the number of people supervising, how food may be distributed, the capabilities to manage meals, the capabilities to manage emergencies, and the like.

In many of these settings, there is no school nurse available, which may add to anxiety. It is certainly possible to create a safe setting, but the challenges are different than for older age groups.

Q: How should parents approach a school to determine the safest routines for their child?
A: The answer to that is "carefully and thoughtfully," with advanced preparation. It's very important for a family to think about the questions they are going to ask and the requests they are going to make prior to actually going to the school. Before making suggestions, it may be wise to first determine what the school has to offer from their prior experience.

For example, some questions families should have in mind ahead of time include:

• Have you ever had children with peanut allergy in your school?

• Specifically, what have you done for them?

• Were there any special problems that arose?

• Do you think your school is safe now for our peanut-allergic child?

• If not, what do you think you could do to assure us that the school will be safe for our child?

By asking questions like these, you can get some ideas about what, if anything, the school has already done to protect allergic children and therefore what they can provide for your child. You may also want to talk to other parents who have food-allergic children in the school. In this way, you will have some vital information regarding your child's safety at the school before you begin introducing any suggestions that may be new, and you will avoid trying to "reinvent the wheel."

I have heard about some schools becoming overwhelmed with a family's lists of requests, particularly if the school had not previously worked with children with peanut allergy. So this suggested approach may avoid confusion or a notion that the school may not be able to provide a safe environment, when they should actually be able to do so.

Q: Are there other specific questions parents should ask the school?
A: Yes. If the school has dealt with allergic children before, you could ask:

• How do you handle meals? For example, do children eat in the classroom or cafeteria?

• How do you handle snacks?

• Who supervises when food is given to the children?

• Which school staff members are trained to recognize allergic reactions and treat them?

• Have you used emergency action plans for children with food allergies, and if so, how have they worked out?

• Do you have experience with allergic children who have had reactions in school, and if so, how have these situations been managed?

• Is there a school nurse? If so, what hours is the nurse at the school?

These and other questions that concern you are helpful starting points so that you and the school can create an effective care plan for your child. If there has been no previous experience with allergic children in the school, additional questions and issues would need to be addressed, and the school would have to not just modify their existing plans for your child, but would have to institute new plans from scratch. Information from this book and The Food Allergy & Anaphylaxis Network will be helpful.

Q: Who should be responsible for the safety of the allergic child?
A: Several organizations, such as the American School Food Service Association, the National Association of Elementary School Principals, the National Association of School Nurses, the National School Board Association, and The Food Allergy & Anaphylaxis Network, got together to define school guidelines for dealing with students with food allergies. (See appendix IV for the full list.)

The bottom line is that the family, the school, and the child all have responsibilities, and by working together, these responsibilities will keep the child safe.

Briefly, the *family's responsibilities* are:

• Providing documentation about the allergy;

• Making sure the medications are available;

• Making sure an emergency action plan is in place; and

• Reviewing the emergency action plan with the school.

The *school's responsibilities* are:

• To understand all the specific ways of protecting the child from ingesting peanut;

• To identify those individuals who are going to be available to supervise and also to treat a problem if it arises; and

• To make sure the people responsible for the child's care have ready access to the emergency action plan and any needed medications.

The *child's responsibilities* are:

• To understand that food cannot be traded with other children;

• Not to eat anything unless he or she definitely knows it is safe; and

• To notify someone immediately if he or she has accidentally eaten anything that may have contained peanut.

Q: What have been some of the major trouble spots for schools handling allergic reactions in their students?
A: In collaboration with The Food Allergy & Anaphylaxis Network, we did a study on reactions that happened in

schools in regard to peanut, and one of the main issues for a lot of the families were reactions that occurred in preschools and child care centers. It seems that for very young children who are not yet in charge of their own bodies, trouble spots arise because they:

• Grab other children's food,

• Pick up crumbs off the floor,

• Lick each other's toys,

and do other similar things that can result in unwanted peanut getting into their mouths. So there is a much greater chance of making a mistake with preschoolers than with grade-school children, who are much more in charge of their bodies and also easier to supervise and unlikely to "lick the table."

Other specific trouble spots also came up in our studies of school reactions. Reactions were categorized by the families as occurring from eating a food with peanut in it; possibly from skin contact with the food, with possible ingestion; and even from smelling the food with possible skin contact or ingestion. In the second two categories, it was not clear whether the child only touched or inhaled the peanut; they may have also actually eaten it.

But a major theme for the ingestion reactions were that in more than half the reactions, the food was a cookie or a bakery product containing peanut that was accidentally ingested. And in almost all the other cases, the food was candy. Less than 10 percent of the time, the child ate a peanut butter sandwich or, in one case, ate chili with peanut, or icing on a cake that had peanut in it.

In regard to the skin contact, possible inhalation, and possible ingestion categories, the overwhelming problem was with *craft projects with peanut*. An example is the pine cone bird feeder made by rubbing peanut butter on pine cones. Consider the scenario: The school knows the child cannot eat peanut, but all twenty children in the classroom are given pine cones and a cup of peanut butter to start smearing peanut on the pine cones. With that amount of peanut all over the tables and hands, it's very easy to have peanut-allergic children touch it, rub it on themselves, or even to accidentally get it into their mouths. Such projects are clearly a poor choice and also exclude the allergic child.

Sometimes schools will use peanut in other craft projects or in a demonstration for science projects, and these are also important issues that have to be considered for schools where there are children who have peanut allergy.

We also found some mistakes that were made when a reaction occurred. Some schools called the family before carrying out the emergency plan, when they should not have delayed treatment to do so. Sometimes symptoms of an allergic reaction were not noticed right away, a mistake that emphasizes the need to review what the symptoms are. In just one case, a school nurse was not familiar with the technique of using the epinephrine injector; while this was a rare problem, it indicates that a discussion about training on the use of the device is important.

Q: What advice do you give in regard to school policies?
A: My advice reflects the advice that is in the list of guidelines already mentioned (see appendix IV) which really boils down to an approach that directly involves the family, school personnel, and child, with additional assistance from the allergist.

There has to be a meeting between the family and

school to identify exactly what has to be done in terms of an emergency plan for the child. That usually boils down to some very simple concepts:

• There should be a physician-directed written emergency plan detailing the treatment of an allergic reaction.

• This emergency plan should be reviewed between the family and the school personnel—for example, a school nurse or an administrator who is going to be in charge of carrying out that plan. It should also be reviewed by any other individuals in the school who will be supervising the child for typical school activities and for mealtimes.

• The emergency plan itself and the medications associated with it should be easily available so that everyone knows where the copies of the plan and the medications themselves are located in the school.

• The medication should not be locked up. People who may need to administer the medications should clearly know how to use them and when to use them, whether nurse, principal, administrator, and/or teacher.

• The school should facilitate keeping the child safe by maintaining a peanut-free food chain. That is, the school should make sure the child is not given foods that contain peanut. This task is also part of the child's or family's responsibilities. It clearly means that there can be no food sharing and that any snacks provided for the allergic child will be peanut-free.

Q: In regard to epinephrine injectors, how many are needed, and where should they be kept?

A: In general, unless the school is in a remote location, two units should be available. However, the school may find it more convenient to have more units for different locations if the school campus is very large. Depending upon local practices and the age of the children, some children may carry their own units. Some schools like to have a unit in the classroom.

To me, the main issue is that one set of injectors should be kept in one unlocked location all the time and known to all, so in the event of an emergency, there are no problems about locating the medication. I am not in favor of passing a unit from teacher to teacher, or student to teacher, as it may become misplaced.

Q: Would it be better for schools just to ban peanuts?
A: Some schools have taken to banning peanuts, with the belief that if everyone is restricted from bringing peanuts to the school, there is less chance for a child with peanut allergy to accidentally eat them. There are certainly arguments on both sides of the fence concerning this issue.

Some people argue that banning peanuts is not a real-life situation for children. They also point out that there are still possibilities for coming across peanut, even if individuals in the school believe they have excluded it, because most people do not understand what avoidance can involve. And there are arguments that it may not be necessary to ban peanuts, because if the children are simply careful not to eat other children's foods, there should not be a problem.

The major argument of the side in favor of banning peanuts is that the mere act of keeping peanuts out of the school is a way to avoid the problem in the first place.

There's probably not a right answer to this question, and what a school decides to do will vary from setting to setting and may vary according to the needs of the child, as well. Some factors that schools may consider include:

• The age, behavior, and maturity of the child;

• Whether belligerence or bullying is an issue; and

• What supervision is available during meals.

I usually suggest that families and schools discuss the options for maximizing safety for the allergic child. Here are two examples of possible outcomes:

1. The family, school principal, nurse, and Robert, a ten-year-old boy with peanut allergy met to discuss options. They established that the school had never banned peanut before and had served it in the cafeteria.

   • Everyone agreed that Robert was not going to share food and would only eat his lunch and snacks from home;
   • There are no belligerent children involved who might try to give Robert peanut on purpose, and if anything like that became an issue, he would tell a teacher; and
   • Robert wanted to eat lunch at a table with his friends.

   The family, student, and school all felt that the best decision was to allow Robert to eat with his friends. The school would explain to the children about Robert's allergy so everyone understood why Robert could not share food.

2. The family of Jenny, a five-year-old girl with peanut allergy, met with the teacher, nurse, lunchroom director,

and principal before Jenny started kindergarten. The children in this school eat in a cafeteria that serves lunch, including peanut, though some children bring their own food from home. The class is split into two tables. During the meeting, it was established that:

• There was one teacher and one aide for two tables;
• The children would likely be messy eaters and could potentially grab another child's food or snack; and
• Jenny was impulsive and had tried to grab snacks from others.

The group felt they could assign one adult to the table where Jenny ate. They would be in the first lunch group, so the table would be clean from the day before. The nurse would prepare a letter asking the children in Jenny's class not to bring in peanut-containing foods for lunch from home, and the cafeteria personnel would not give peanut to this class. The teacher would sit at the table with Jenny and reinforce "no food sharing," teaching her this concept. After lunch, the children would wash up before coming back to their classroom.

Q: So, while some schools may ban peanut, others may restrict peanut in certain places?
A: Yes. Another solution that some schools use is what is called a "peanut-free" or "allergy" table. The compromise here is that although peanut is not excluded from everyone in the class or in the cafeteria, there is a table where the peanut-allergic children can select friends who are not eating peanut-containing meals to sit with them. In that way, everyone sitting at that particular table eats a peanut-free meal, and the table becomes a safe environment where

there are fewer issues about food sharing or accidental exposures. Still, no food is shared.

Q: What if the allergic child does not like the idea of a "peanut-free" table?
A: While many schools have used the compromise of a peanut-free table, particularly as children get older, many children do not like to be segregated in this way. While this is an issue that should certainly be discussed with your physician, I do not see a problem for most of my patients with having older children sitting at a regular table, as long as they know not to share food with the other children and just eat their own food that is safe.

Q: What about parties? Wouldn't this leave out the child with peanut allergies?
A: Strict "no food sharing" policies are a primary way to avoid problems, and our studies show that school parties are a trouble spot. If there is any notion that the child would take food provided by others, it puts the responsibility of label reading or safe food preparation on people who are not living with food allergy and may not have the required information to provide safe foods.

It's difficult enough for families with allergic children to understand how to read labels and make sure that all the foods consumed are safe. So it is particularly hard to expect families who are not living with issues of peanut avoidance to create safe food options. Therefore, in many cases, it is unrealistic and unsafe to expect safe foods in these situations. For many families, I suggest having a box of ready-to-eat snacks available so if there's a party, then the child who has peanut allergy can simply take one of those snacks as an alternative.

Some families of peanut-allergic children will actually provide snacks for the whole class at times. By doing so, they know the food being eaten is peanut-safe for their own children. There are also schools where the cafeteria personnel are adequately trained to create peanut-free meals and can also provide food for parties. Therefore, if you discuss these kinds of preparations with the school, and everyone feels they are well-educated in providing peanut-free foods, it's quite possible to rely on the school for food for celebrations, as well.

Q: What are the most important points to emphasize to children old enough to take some responsibility for their peanut allergy?
A: In regard to studies on reactions in schools and poor outcomes, I would emphasize no food sharing and understanding and following a prescribed emergency action plan, which means notifying an adult of any problems such as symptoms of a reaction, so epinephrine can be injected promptly if needed.

Q: What is an "emergency action plan" for a school?
A: In my view, an emergency action plan really includes a wide array of points. This plan is usually a written agreement that identifies:

• The child,

• The allergy and the symptoms that may be experienced,

• The medications that will be given in the event of an exposure or reaction, and

• Telephone numbers for reaching medical care and for contacting the family.

This action plan is a component of an overall peanut-allergy care plan. Such a plan extends to issues beyond the written emergency action plan to make sure that the child, the family, and school personnel are all on the same page in regard to:

• How peanut is going to be avoided for that child;

• Who will be responsible for supervising to insure that peanut is not ingested;

• Who will make sure that those supervising the child will be able to recognize an allergic reaction and respond appropriately; and

• What action will be taken in the event of an exposure or reaction, which should be reviewed carefully from start to finish, in terms of what could actually happen in such an emergency situation.

I think it's useful for the school to think about the precise chain of command in case of an accidental ingestion or reaction. For example, if a child accidentally ate a cookie that contained peanut and started to break out in hives:

• Who would take the child to the school nurse?

• Who would administer medications if the school nurse was not there?

• Or if there is no school nurse, who is in charge of administering the medications to the child?

• Who will contact emergency services, such as 911?

All these actions need to be clearly spelled out in advance, both in writing and in discussions, so if an emergency occurs, no one will have any doubts about what to do, and no time will be wasted in getting help for the allergic child. I suggest that parents review these actions with the school in advance. In addition, the emergency plan should be periodically reviewed to make sure that the personnel in charge of recognizing and treating the allergic reactions are still in place; and also to make sure that any required medications are kept up to date and have not expired. Periodic review, like a fire drill, can also refresh everyone's memory of the plan and identify any shortcomings.

Q: What do allergic children and their families have to be aware of in terms of travel on the school bus?
A: Bus trips to school and back are anxiety-producing for many families, because there is not the same type of supervision on the bus that there is in school. An important suggestion in regard to the bus is not to have any parties on the bus involving food.

In addition, younger children with peanut allergies can sit at the front of the bus near the driver, so they can be observed to make sure that they are not sharing food or eating any food. Some families request that their allergic children be picked up at a point in the bus route that is as close as possible to the school to shorten the trip if possible, and they also advise the bus driver about locations of hospitals or emergency clinics, and the emergency action plans, just in case there is a problem with an allergic reaction on the bus.

Q: What do people need to know about school trips?
A: This is another area where advance preparation is key. Depending upon the nature of the trip, tips that are applicable to travel and vacations may apply (see chapter 28) When there is a school trip, the emergency action plan may need to be reviewed with different people than usual, depending upon who will be on the trip. Bringing safe foods and snacks along will avoid issues that arise in restaurant eating (see chapter 26) that may be too complicated to undertake for inexperienced chaperones.

So when it comes to school trips for children with peanut allergies, most families try to make sure there is an extremely safe meal, such as a bagged lunch, already available for their allergic children. In that way, the allergic children are not dependent upon getting their food in a restaurant setting. Also, the medications the children need for an allergic reaction are carried along on the trip, and there are adults present, monitoring the children, who understand the emergency plan in regard to identifying a reaction and responding appropriately.

Q: Should children with peanut allergies ever eat food supplied by a school?
A: The answer is "yes," but only if they are certain that the school is able to provide a safe meal. Whether the school can or cannot do that is something that the family has to discuss with appropriate school staff members. The exact same rules and educational process that families go

through in learning how to provide a safe meal for their child have to be reviewed with the school. They need to understand:

• Issues of cross-contact,

• How to read food labels, and

• How to be certain that the food they provide for allergic children is free from peanut or peanut contamination.

If both school and family are confident that all this can be clearly understood and accomplished, then there is no reason why allergic children should not eat food supplied by the school.

Q: Do children with peanut allergies have any special legal rights in a school?
A: They do, although in my experience, it is rarely necessary to invoke legal plans to establish a safe school program. Most schools are eager to insure that your child is safe and to work with you on an allergy care plan/emergency action plan that is effective.

The Americans with Disabilities Act, Title Three, indicates that "no individual shall be discriminated against on the basis of disability in the full and equal enjoyment of the goods and services of any public accommodation." The Rehabilitation Act of 1973, Section 504, Public Law 93-112 prohibits discrimination in education on the basis of handicap in any program or institution receiving federal funds. Usually, this law is applied for people with educational problems, such as those with learning disabilities, visual impairments, or deafness. If you are disabled, there are many obvious factors that can interrupt your ability to have a successful experience at school unless there is some intervention.

But the same law also applies to children with other medical problems, such as seizures, diabetes, or peanut allergies. It is possible to set up a "504 plan" that essentially says that if you have a disability, the school must put together a care plan that makes it possible for you to attend school safely and effectively, even with your disability. So this law is one way of insuring that:

• There is an emergency action plan in place, and

• Substitutes for peanuts are used in the school setting.

As stated above, I rarely have had parents set up this legal document, because most schools set up emergency action plans without problems. But let's say staff members at a school want to use peanuts for a lesson in counting objects with young children and just refuse to substitute anything else, even though your child is allergic. You have explained your concern, but the school is obstinate. If the school receives federal funds, you can use a 504 plan to compel the school substitute pennies for peanuts in the counting exercise.

Q: Are there any special issues for attending college?
A: There are actually numerous issues for college-age people with peanut allergy. As indicated elsewhere in this book, this is an age group at particular risk, because eating dangerously becomes more common, and denial of symptoms with delayed medical treatment is an addi-

tional problem. On top of these, experimentation with alcohol or drugs can impair judgment and increase risks. The problems are possibly compounded, as the student may be away from his or her usual support network. So it's particularly important with this college-age group to discuss and emphasize safety issues in order to make sure that no risks are being taken and that the peers of the student, as well as the health center of the college, know about the allergy. In that way, if anything happens, the allergic person will be able to get help from those who are with him or her.

In college, there is an additional issue: Most college students are not going to bring food from home with them every day and are instead going to depend on getting most of their meals in a cafeteria setting. Because of this, families should meet with the food services personnel in the college to discuss the allergy, even ahead of any final decisions about attendance. Many of these food services have experienced food allergy issues before, but the families will still want to confirm with them exactly what is available to their college-age student in that particular school setting in regard to a safe meal. The bottom line is that the food service personnel need to understand how to create a meal that is peanut-free, and families must make sure that everyone understands what is involved and feels comfortable that a safe meal can be provided. The dining services personnel must understand the issues of label reading and cross-contact. Advance preparation is the key. And many of the same day-to-day rules of living with a food allergy are going to apply even more strictly with someone who is living in a college setting.

The school guidelines (see appendix IV) indicate that there are responsibilities for students to keep themselves

safe. I am a firm believer that families should always partner with their children, even from a young age, to share responsibilities for their peanut allergy. This teaches children
how to keep themselves safe during a time when there is
adult supervision and therefore provides children with the
tools they need to obtain safe meals and take care of themselves when they finally "leave the nest."

Case History

JOHN

John, a five-year-old with peanut allergy and asthma,
was going to start school in the fall. His parents had already approached a private school, which said they could
not accept him because his allergy could not be managed
by their staff. The parents then decided they wanted to
send their son to the local public school, but they wanted
the school to ban peanuts. They came to see me for advice about how they could handle this situation.

After some discussion, I discovered that John's family
had presented the private school with a twenty-page
book of instructions they had prepared, detailing everything they expected the school to do to keep peanuts
away from John. It included having everyone wash their
hands frequently and clean the rooms and furniture often, and specified exactly what the other children could
and could not do. Their emergency action plan was several pages long, and the book stated that if John was even
near peanut, he would likely die.

Obviously, this book must have been overwhelming to
the private school, which would have had to change almost all their routines in order to accommodate John. Al-

though there are many concerns that families should have when their children attend school, the issues need to be presented in a way that makes it possible for the family and school to work together in a reasonable way to insure a child's safety.

We talked about John's ability to protect himself, which was not very good for a five-year-old. We discussed the routines at school that would make the family comfortable, and whether or not peanuts had to be totally banned from the premises. We also talked about how they could approach the school by meeting with them ahead of time and reviewing the school's experiences with other allergic children and how they had insured their safety in the past.

Feeling more confident about what to do, John's family talked to the school and discovered that they had a full-time school nurse, that in her absence there was a person designated and trained to handle emergencies, and the school also had had two other children with peanut allergy in their kindergarten classes recently who had been fine. In this school, the children ate lunch in their classrooms, and the school had requested no-peanut lunches in the specific classrooms where the peanut-allergic children were present.

For added insurance, the family asked me to talk to the school, and I reviewed some of the major issues, such as not using peanuts for classroom activities, including cooking projects; that there should be a frequently reviewed "no food sharing" policy; how parties should be handled; and how the children's hands could be cleaned and the tables cleaned after lunch. With John's emergency action plan in place, a school nurse present, and an unlocked storage area for his medications, the family was reassured, and John went on to have a successful year in his new school, with no allergic problems.

Case History

JIM

At seventeen years of age, Jim was getting ready for college. He came to see me with his parents, who were very concerned about Jim's ability to protect himself without the supervision of his family. Although he had only had a couple of accidental exposures to peanut over his lifetime, Jim's peanut allergy was a major concern for them because he didn't seem to be taking his peanut allergy and asthma very seriously.

Since he would be away from home, the family had checked out prospective colleges to be sure that the cafeterias could provide Jim with safe meals. They had confirmed with me that Jim had not outgrown his peanut allergy and knew he could be at risk of a severe reaction if he accidentally ingested peanut, because he had both asthma and a peanut allergy. Since Jim had been watched over by his parents his entire life, he had not experienced dealing with food allergy for himself, which was now a major concern. At college, Jim would have a whole new group of friends who would not be familiar with his allergies and might not look out for him the way his current friends always had. Jim's parents felt he needed to understand the seriousness of the new situation he was facing, so he would not be careless about possible exposure to peanut.

After discussing the college situation with the family, I took Jim aside to talk to him alone. We know from studies that teenagers with peanut allergy and asthma are at the highest risk for fatal reactions, largely because their behavior is often more risky, and they may not treat themselves promptly if they have a reaction. And because the family told me that Jim was downplaying his allergy, I knew it was possible that he might be at additional risk.

I was also aware that when Jim was on his own at college, he would most likely be exposed to both alcohol and drugs, and if he used them, that could further increase his risks, since they affect your ability to monitor yourself and make good judgments, for example, about dietary choices and when medication might be needed.

So we discussed the fact that Jim's condition was a serious one, that he had to become independent of his parents but also demonstrate that he could assume responsibility for himself, that he had to make good judgments that would protect his health, and that he needed to tell his new friends about his allergies. We reviewed how important it was for him to discuss the allergies with his friends; how he was older and more responsible and could begin and continue to introduce the issue of peanut allergy when dining out, to insure a safe meal. We discussed the importance of always having medications available, and we reviewed how and why they would be used. We even discussed dating and issues of kissing if his partner had eaten peanut.

Jim and I made a short written agreement that he would do these things and let me or his family know if he was having trouble. I gave him some printed material from The Food Allergy & Anaphylaxis Network about teenagers with allergies to back up the discussion. I instructed his family to give him more "practice time" to take charge of his allergies and to monitor how he was doing in the months ahead before college. As a result, Jim's transition to college was far less stressful for the family, and Jim seemed to have a better grasp of his role in assuming greater responsibility for his health and well-being.

25.

Summer Camps

Q: Is the approach to peanut allergy different in camps, as compared to schools?

A: The approach for a camp setting is almost identical to the approach for a school setting. However, there are a few issues that make camps a little more difficult in terms of insuring safety.

One issue is that you may have younger supervisors at a camp. In a school setting the teacher is usually an adult who can understand and carry out emergency plans and prevent allergic children from getting into trouble in the first place, perhaps more effectively than a teenage counselor in a camp setting would be able to do. Many camps have nurses, and since they are usually the people who direct the emergency plans, this issue is not usually a problem.

The other issue that comes up with camps is that there may be frequent field trips, which carry the same pitfalls that field trips do in school settings.

Overnight camps are yet another issue for those with a peanut allergy, because in that type of camp, meals are being provided for the allergic child, rather than just lunch or snacks at a day camp. So families need to discuss and think about all of these issues as they select a camp.

Q: What should families look for when they select a camp?
A: To address the same concerns that arise for schools, and the additional ones that arise for camps, the issues to be considered will include:

• The number and origin of meals and snacks,

• The supervision available during meals,

• Whether there is a camp nurse,

• What provisions have been made in the past for children with peanut allergies,

• Who would be responsible for managing and carrying out an emergency action plan,

• What the procedures are for travel and trips,

• What training could be or has been provided in regard to allergy for people supervising meals and trips,

• What the situation would be if a reaction occurred, and

• What hospitals services are available.

As described for schools (see chapter 24), preparation is key, and meeting with the camp director in advance would be an important start. Assuming you are comfortable with the camp's capabilities, more specific instructions can be reviewed. There is a spectrum of possible issues that may arise in these conversations. You'll need to decide whether or not the camp is right for your child in regard to meal provisions and snacks. If it's a day camp, and the allergic children are bringing their own food, that eliminates a lot of these problems. But if they're not, will this camp be able to provide a safe lunch or, in some cases, three meals plus snacks? There are camps that are able to do this, but a lot of discussion has to be undertaken to insure safety. You will also need to consider the camp's capabilities to set up the same type of emergency action plan that schools follow.

Q: Is it possible for children with peanut allergies to go to sleep-away camp?
A: Going away to camp carries additional stress. For many families, having their peanut-allergic children at a distance seems almost unimaginable. Even so, I have patients who go to sleep-away camps. But it takes significant preparation on the part of the family in regard to insuring that the camp can manage the peanut allergy from all the same perspectives that have been previously discussed.

For example, the camp may be at a distance from a hospital, which can provide an additional source of anxiety. So it's important for the camp to have a clear-cut emergency plan in place and to have an acceptable way to get allergic children to medical care if they need it.

Q: How close should the camp be to a hospital?
A: This is certainly a judgment call, and issues of the specific camp and your own comfort level will weigh in to the decision. On the one hand, you do not want your peanut-

allergic child to have a reaction when he or she is in a re-mote location and unable to get to medical care. On the other hand, you do not want to exclude a superb camp just because a hospital is not one block away. This same issue also comes up in deciding where to go on vacation.

You would probably only feel comfortable with a camp that has very reasonable measures in place to insure your child's safety in the first place. Therefore, the major concern here regards activation of emergency services. You should discuss this issue specifically with the camp director and/or nurse. Camps have to manage any of a number of medical emergencies—for example, children with medical problems such as seizures—or they have to care for a child in the event of an injury or allergic reaction to an insect sting, and they can likely explain their procedures to you.

Some seemingly small measures may provide reassurance. For example, walkie-talkies for hikes or cell phones for trips would expedite access to care. Of course, the main line of safety is the overall care plan to avoid peanut ingestion and the emergency action plan to provide treatments in the event of an accidental ingestion, to reduce the risk of a problem in the first place. You, your child, the camp personnel, and your allergist should all feel comfortable with the provisions so that the camp experience is an enjoyable one.

26

Restaurants and Food Services

Q: Do restaurants have sufficient information and expertise about food allergies?
A: While many restaurants have some knowledge about food allergies, it's probably safer for consumers to assume that they know very little about food allergies.

Q: What are some of the common pitfalls for people who eat in restaurants and have peanut allergies?
A: We did a study on this question from among those in our registry of people with peanut allergies maintained in conjunction with The Food Allergy & Anaphylaxis Network. Reactions and errors resulted from mistakes on the side of both the allergic individual and the restaurants. In regard to consumers, it seems that the biggest pitfall is *lack of communication to the restaurant staff that the adult or child has an actual allergy, rather than just a distaste for peanut.*

For example, just asking if there is peanut in a particular dish on the menu does not necessarily imply to the restaurant personnel that you are concerned that even a small amount of peanut might cause a life-threatening reaction. In other words, they may be less likely to truly consider the specific intention of your request.

Conversely, if you say to a restaurant, "I or my child is highly peanut-allergic; even a tiny amount could cause a serious health risk or reaction," they are going to look at the meal with more care in regard to the risk that there is peanut in the food.

One risk that applies to most types of restaurants is that your server may not know the actual ingredients of the food. Sometimes a server assumes that he or she knows the ingredients but does not. There are also instances of cross-contact of the final meal with peanut, which can happen in the kitchen. This is particularly an issue for Asian restaurants and for dessert items in various restaurants.

Q: Does that mean certain restaurants are more dangerous?
A: Based upon our studies, the restaurants or food services that seem to cause the most problems for peanut-allergic people include:

• Asian restaurants,

• Bakeries, and

• Ice cream parlors or ice cream-dessert restaurants.

Even if you're in one of these places and are ordering food that does not have peanut as a specific ingredient, whether it's ice cream, a bakery-type dessert, or beef and broccoli in a Chinese restaurant, all these foods could be cross-contaminated with peanut during preparation in that particular restaurant's kitchen and are therefore a higher risk.

Q: What other pitfalls have you seen?
A: There can be problems with salad bars or serve-yourself buffets. Sometimes there are peanuts in some dishes, and people may spill them from one tray to the next or use the same serving spoons and introduce peanut into foods where there was no peanut before.

Q: In regard to ice cream parlors, what if the server washes out the scoop before serving?
A: There are a number of issues in ice cream shops. The thought about washing the scoop is that any peanut from a previous serving could be washed off before your vanilla is scooped. However, imagine that the person before you ordered a double scoop with peanut ripple and vanilla. The peanut from the first swipe may have been carried into the vanilla. Now your server has a clean scooper, but it does not matter, because the vanilla ice cream is already contaminated. In other words, washing the scoop does not hurt, but it does not eliminate risks. Another issue in the ice cream shop is the toppings. Peanut could get spilled into nonpeanut toppings.

Q: What are some of the specific problems that arise in restaurants?
A: There are several trouble spots. Many of the problems in restaurants are the same basic problems that you have when shopping for yourself or your peanut-allergic child. For ex-

ample, they may be using some premanufactured products, so the restaurant staff would have to look carefully at the labels to make sure that peanut is not an ingredient.

At the next level, peanut may be an ingredient in a food, but not as whole peanuts. For example, the dish could contain peanut flour or peanut oil, and these could end up in the food without there being any actual solid or visible peanuts included. Many times, the restaurant staff and even the peanut-allergic person or family may not think about peanuts if they don't actually see them, and that's trouble.

A sad example is a fatal incident that occurred in a restaurant many years ago when someone who was peanut-allergic ordered chili. In this particular restaurant, peanuts were an ingredient used to thicken and flavor the chili, even though they could not be seen, and the consumer had a severe reaction and died before medical help could be obtained.

In the same way, peanut flour might be used to flavor or thicken certain food products, or peanut oil or even peanut butter might be used to thicken a variety of sauces or foods. In these cases, again, you don't see any actual peanuts in the foods, and you might mistakenly assume they are safe.

Another problem is cross-contact of a safe food with peanut. For example, some restaurants may stock peanuts in small dishes for use on bar or buffet areas, so some peanut may get into the food being prepared for the allergic person. In a bakery or restaurant, even if peanut is not a specific ingredient, there may be grinders, utensils, mixing bowls, and other equipment that may have been used for peanut, and peanut residue could get into a food that doesn't contain any peanut as an ingredient. In Asian restaurants, you may order beef and broccoli, but it may have been made in the exact same wok that one meal before had peanut in it. So these are all important issues that a restaurant has to deal with in providing a safe meal.

Q: Can you provide some additional examples of restaurant problems with hidden ingredients and cross-contact that have actually happened?
A: Some examples of incidents I have learned about in my practice, through studies we've done, and in the literature include:

• A piecrust had peanut embedded in it, so you couldn't actually see the nuts.

• An ice cream cone had a face on it made from small chocolate-covered candies, and one of them had peanut in it. The family asked if the candies contained peanut, and the salesperson said, "Oh no, those are just chocolate," but they turned out to be chocolate-covered peanut candies.

• Egg roll was sealed with peanut butter or, in another situation, had peanut flour in it.

• A garnish in a salad had finely chopped peanuts.

• A jelly sandwich, just like the kind that can be made in the home, was contaminated with peanut, because the jelly had previously been used for a peanut butter and jelly sandwich.

• Ice cream scoopers had been used to serve peanut-containing ice cream.

• A server had sprinkled peanuts on another dessert and still had some peanuts on his hands when he was preparing food for a peanut-allergic person.

Q: How should peanut-allergic patrons discuss their allergies with restaurant staff?
A: Most important is that the main starting point is to make it clear that you or your child has *a life-threatening peanut allergy, not just a dislike for peanuts*.

The Food Allergy & Anaphylaxis Network suggests what's called "chef's cards," and examples are available on their Web site (see resources). They are a list of what the person is allergic to, if they're allergic to multiple things. But for peanut-specific allergies, the card should include wording that specifically describes the allergy, such as "I or my child is allergic to peanut. Even a small amount could cause a serious problem. Here are some examples of items that may contain peanut. What I need is to make sure that this restaurant understands that any food we order can not have even the smallest amount of peanut in it. We need to feel confident that your restaurant can provide us with a safe meal." Then a list of risky foods can follow.

The next step involves making sure there is a good line of communication between you and the people making and serving the food. What that usually means is that the person preparing the meal should come out and discuss what is involved in the creation of the meal with the peanut-allergic person or family. After that discussion, you should be able to order foods that, presumably, would be quite safe.

For example, a tuna fish sandwich on toast doesn't sound like it would likely contain peanut, but you still need to get assurance from the restaurant that it will not.

Some of the problems that come up when allergic reactions occur in restaurants are partly because the consumer assumes that some foods would have to be safe, by virtue of the type of foods that they are. But you have to remember that you never know if someone has cross-contaminated the food or has put in some "secret" ingredient, and it is not worth the risk to assume. So it's always worthwhile not to be embarrassed, to really discuss the peanut allergy, and to never make any assumptions.

Also remember that you should always talk to the restaurant staff member who really understands what is in the food. Sometimes that's conveyed through a waiter, but usually it involves a manager or the chef or the kitchen worker who is preparing the actual meal.

So to summarize the question about how peanut-allergic patrons should discuss their allergies with a restaurant, the answer would be to describe them in very specific detail, possibly with written backup. And after the meal comes to the table, they should have a confirming discussion just to be absolutely certain that the food is safe and does not contain peanut.

Peanut-allergic people should probably not even be ordering foods that are "riskier" and could pose a problem. So it's probably better to pick a fruit dessert rather than a brownie. Also be careful about the types of restaurants you're choosing to eat in. It would take a tremendous amount of discussion to make sure that you have a safe meal in an Asian restaurant. It is not impossible, but it would just take a lot more effort. You would have to really make sure that you can rely on the people you're speaking to and that they clearly understand everything you're saying, since peanut is so often found in their menu items. If, for any restaurant, you try to obtain a safe meal and do not feel confident that you have succeeded, don't eat the food!

Q: How can you be assured that your meal is safe?
A: The answer to this requires your own judgment based upon your interactions at the restaurant. Mistakes or accidents can occur, but you have to do your very best and attain a level of comfort that is reasonable for you. This should certainly be attainable in most circumstances. You want to make sure that:

• The line of communication between you and the restaurant staff is as clear as possible.

• The foods you order are not high-risk foods or in high-risk settings as described above.

• If you have a gut feeling that the people you spoke with don't really understand what the situation is, then you should not take a chance and eat the food. Instead, you should just walk out and eat elsewhere.

Q: If an allergic reaction does occur in a restaurant, what should be done?
A: There have been some terrible mistakes in regard to action taken at restaurants. You certainly should use your medications and make sure you have them with you at all times. Some of the worst outcomes in restaurants were simply because food-allergic people did not have their medications with them. The restaurants don't have them, of course, so you must always carry your medication with you.

There have also been bad outcomes where the restaurant staff asked allergic people to leave because they were having reactions and it was frightening the other patrons.

What you really want to do is make sure that you follow your plan to use the appropriate emergency medications, that *911 is called immediately* and told that a severe allergic reaction is taking place, and that emergency care arrives, and everything in the person's emergency plan is followed.

Q: Are there circumstances you can describe where you may not be comfortable about eating in a particular restaurant?
A: Again, this is a judgment call, but I can give some examples.

If someone ever makes a mistake and, for example, a salad comes out with nuts on top, you may well not feel comfortable eating anything in that restaurant. But if you decide that you are going to stay and eat, instead of sending the salad back, you should say to the server, "We just talked about making sure there would not be any nuts in my food, and here are nuts. I'm going to hold on to this dish. I need to have a new one made that you can assure me does not have peanut in it."

The reason for holding on to that dish is that there have been reactions from the restaurant staff just removing whatever the person is allergic to, and thinking that is good enough, even though small amounts of the offending food remain. Just picking off the nuts or taking off the top layer is obviously not good enough.

If the server seemed disinterested in your description of your allergy, or seemed to be brushing it off, you should probably leave. Also, if the person who made the food is not available and there is no way to get food for which someone knows the ingredients, you should leave.

Q: Are allergic issues being addressed from the side of the restaurant?

A: There are many potential loose ends in restaurant food preparation that could cause problems for people with allergies, as discussed above. Currently, there are no comprehensive required training programs or rules for dealing with food allergy in food service locations. One of the problems is that many restaurants have a big worker turnover, and so you don't necessarily know the experience levels of those who are providing your meals. That's why, at this time, a lot of the burden falls on consumers to make sure that they have discussed the issues appropriately and received reasonable assurance that the people preparing their meals understand what the issues are and can provide safe meals.

New guidelines for food services are coming into place soon, with more educational issues regarding food allergy, including the notion that peanut is a very important allergen and that cross-contact can occur in a variety of ways in a restaurant setting and can cause serious problems. The Food Allergy & Anaphylaxis Network and the Food Allergy Initiative, with input from various restaurant and food service organizations, have created guidance programs regarding food allergy for restaurants and food services. So this issue is something that will become a part of the education of food providers. But at this point in time, it can't be depended upon, since most restaurants have not provided training.

One thought is that restaurants could provide ingredients lists on their menus. I am not so certain that this would ever become a full solution, but for now, I would not assume such lists of meal descriptions should be trusted. Even if you see a menu that has an ingredients list with each meal, you should not assume that there is no peanut just because it's not listed there. You still have to engage in a full discussion with the restaurant staff.

Case History

VICTORIA

Victoria's family liked to eat out in restaurants quite often. However, when Victoria, the youngest of three children and the only one with a peanut allergy, had two allergic reactions to peanut in her first few years of life, her parents decided to stop taking their children out to eat with them. As a result, the entire family was unhappy, with her siblings blaming Victoria for not being able to eat out with their parents and Victoria feeling guilty and punished.

The family came to see me to find out if there was something that could be done to solve this problem. We reviewed the allergic reactions Victoria had experienced in the past. One was in an ice cream dessert restaurant where the parents had asked all the right questions. Victoria had an ice cream cone with a clown face on it that the waiter said was made of chocolate. It turned out to have peanut butter in it instead, and Victoria had an allergic reaction. Her second reaction occurred in a Chinese restaurant, where she had eaten before without a problem. This time, however, Victoria ate an egg roll that turned out to contain peanut flour; in addition, peanut butter had been used to seal it. After these two bad experiences eating out, the family was fearful of taking Victoria to any other restaurants.

In our discussion, her parents realized that both situations occurred in high-risk food situations, namely, an ice cream parlor and an Asian restaurant. I discussed with them that with additional education and perhaps safer restaurant choices, they could significantly reduce the risks of a reaction. I suggested that they should avoid bakeries, ice cream parlors, and Asian restaurants. Next, they should talk to the people who actually prepare the food, such as the chefs, since waiters may not know what ingredients have been used to prepare the food. They also have to make sure the person they are speaking to and the one who is preparing the food understand the dangers of cross-contact and that Victoria has a serious allergy, not just a dislike for peanut.

After this visit, Victoria's family understood that by following all these protective procedures, they would be able to take Victoria and their other children out to eat together and that Victoria could indeed receive a safe meal.

27.

Friends' Homes, Play Dates, and Sitters

Q: Should peanut-allergic people be aware of anything special in regard to eating at a friend's or relative's house, as compared to a restaurant?
A: Many of the same rules are going to apply in terms of eating outside the home, whether it's at a school, a friend's house, or a restaurant. There must be an understanding that:

• Even a very small amount of peanut can cause a problem,

• There are certain foods that are particularly high-risk, and

• There are issues with cross-contact.

All these issues have to be considered when someone with a peanut allergy goes to a friend's house. But there are some ways to avoid these problems to begin with.

For example, provide a snack or bagged lunch ahead of time for the allergic child to take to the friend's or relative's house. When you do that, issues of having someone who does not have to live with peanut allergy prepare a safe meal for this child don't even have to come up, as long as no other food in the house is eaten.

Q: What else can be done before eating at a friend's or relative's home?
A: If it's possible for you or your child to bring your own food to someone else's house, that is probably the simplest and easiest way to avoid any bad outcomes. However, there may be situations, especially at relatives' homes, when meals are being prepared for the family and the child for celebrations and for holidays, and you might not feel comfortable bringing your own food. In these situations, for social and practical reasons, the allergic person is going to be eating food prepared by someone who is not living with peanut allergy.

All of the same educational issues are going to arise here, so it's going to be important and hopefully well-received to discuss all the nuances of making a peanut-free meal with your friends or relatives. The same issues of cross-contact and reading labels need to be thoroughly discussed and probably supervised or double-checked by you. If you feel confident that your friends or relatives can give appropriate attention to these issues and understand what they're doing, then you will probably feel comfortable eating their food. But if there is any doubt, it's always safer to avoid any potentially problematic meals.

Q: What do peanut-allergic people need to know about birthday parties?
A: One of the biggest hurdles faced by the families of children with peanut allergies are the continuous invitations to

birthday parties, where unsafe birthday cake and many other snacks that may contain peanut are going to be served.

What many families do is provide substitute snack foods for their children, so the children can go to the party, participate in the games and other activities, and when it comes time for actually eating, they have a safe meal that is already prepared for them.

Some families call ahead to the family giving the birthday party to find out exactly what foods and snacks they will be providing. In this way, the family is sometimes able to provide a meal for their allergic child that looks very similar or exactly the same as the one the other children are eating.

Q: For a play date, is it necessary to completely educate the caretaker about the child's allergy, including the self-injectable epinephrine?
A: I believe that the answer to this is "yes," even when the play date does not involve food. It's always better to be safe than sorry, and although sometimes it might possibly cause some anxiety for the person who is taking your child into their home, it could still be done in a way that does not make the situation seem overwhelming. Some families avoid play dates altogether, and others have tried to educate their hosts, but sometimes this has been met with concern and withdrawal of the invitation. I think patience and persistence should prevail to allow the child with a peanut allergy to enjoy play dates in a safe environment. Even though a parent without a food-allergic child may at first be worried about the self-injectable epinephrine and potential for a reaction, with time and instruction, the anxiety should be allayed. There are many ways to make play dates less stressful.

For example, if children are bringing their own food to a

play date and they are old enough where they are unlikely to indiscriminately take food from other children or other locations, then there is very little reason to be concerned about any problems that could occur during the play date. If food is being provided by the host family, it may be worthwhile to review what will be given. For instance, you could look over some prepackaged snacks and approve or not approve their safety. If a meal is being made from scratch, more instruction would be needed—almost like a restaurant meal.

In regard to the epinephrine, it is safest, and a good habit, to review a copy of the emergency action plan; show your host how to use the self-injectable device and describe when to use it. This is probably the most anxiety-producing aspect of the play date, but you can emphasize that it is highly unlikely that the medicine would be needed as long as the food is safe. You will want to leave contact numbers, as well. Of course, if your child has asthma and is symptomatic, it may make sense to defer a play date, because it can become confusing for the host if your child is coughing and wheezing.

The questions of safety should be discussed with the family taking your child, so that they feel comfortable. Some families of allergic children stay in the house for a play date, either for a little while or for one entire play date, just to see how things go. If all goes well, then for play dates after that, everyone is always more comfortable when the allergic child is in the friend's house on his or her own.

Q: What is your advice when parents leave their child in their own home under the care of another person?
A: All of the issues discussed in this chapter certainly apply to persons providing care for your peanut-allergic child

in your home, such as babysitters or nannies. Specifically, do not assume your food is safe, and carefully review your emergency action plan with the caregiver. You should:

• Review what safe foods are available in the house;

• Make sure the caregiver is fully aware of the allergy;

• Review your emergency action plan in detail with the caregiver, including all the symptoms of a reaction and the treatments that should be given; and

• Review how to activate emergency services and provide the contact numbers to reach help.

Case History

CASEY

An active boy, Casey was seven years old and enjoyed playing with his friend, Alex. But because of Casey's peanut allergy, Alex always came to Casey's house for play dates. Recently, Casey had begun asking his parents if he could go to play at Alex's house. The problem was that Alex's mother was terrified of having Casey in her home, since she felt she would not be able to cope if he had an allergic reaction.

So when Casey's family came to see me, their main questions were, "How do we deal with play dates so that other families are not so worried? Should we tell them about epinephrine? Should we just tell them not to give him anything to eat?"

In our discussion, I told Casey's family that it seemed a fine goal to have him play at other children's homes, but they should also understand why other people feel nervous about having a child with peanut allergy in their homes when they haven't had any previous experience with this situation. I suggested that they begin by having Casey's mother explain about the allergy, but also stay for the first one or two play dates at Alex's house, so she could monitor the situation and explain to Alex's mother how to protect Casey.

While at the house, Casey's mother could show Alex's mother how to use the self-injectable epinephrine device and also reassure her that since Casey will not be eating any of their food, the likelihood of his having an allergic reaction is extremely low. However, she should explain that, for safety, she likes Casey to always have his medication with him, even if the chance of a reaction is virtually zero. Casey would also bring along his own, safe food for a snack, so Alex's mother would not have to worry about his foods or making an error.

Casey's mother followed through on this advice, and Casey began to enjoy play dates with his friend in Alex's home, where Alex's mother was far more comfortable and at ease with having Casey there.

28

Vacations

Q: Is there such a thing as a "safe" vacation?
A: You should be able to arrange a vacation that is safe and enjoyable. I tell my patients and their families that they can enjoy vacations by following many of the same cautions that they set up for day-to-day living. The extra challenge of vacations, of course, is that in most circumstances, you're going to depend on others to provide your food. So all the issues that come up with restaurant eating, for instance, are also going to be part and parcel of dealing with vacations. In addition, advance preparation will be needed.

While there may not be a specific "safe" vacation, some options are probably easier than others. For example, travel to a foreign country where you cannot speak the native language would be more challenging than travel to a local resort that has experience with making safe meals and perhaps offers some options for you to make some meals on your own.

You may feel more secure at a resort near a hospital rather than on a cruise with difficult access to medical care.

There are numerous variables to consider and weigh against your own circumstances, but you want to consider all of these issues in advance so when it is time for vacation, you have very little stress and plenty of time for enjoyment.

Q: What specific preparations should be taken before a vacation?
A: I generally advise my patients to think about their vacation plans with an eye toward day-to-day issues that may arise in regard to their food allergy. For example:

• How are they going to get there?

• Where are they going to be staying in between home and their destination?

• Where are they going to be staying during the vacation?

• How long are they going to be there?

• Where are their meals going to come from?

• What would happen if an allergic reaction occurred?

These are all questions that you need to answer to the best extent possible before you go, so there will not be any unwanted surprises. When you are about to leave, make sure you have all of your medications, know how to access emergency care, have your written allergy plans and possibly written instructions for restaurants, and whatever "backup" foods you need. Since you may be taking meals out frequently, you may want to bring along wet wipes to clean off tables, seats, and high chairs. You want to be able to relax during your vacation and not worry about anything, and advance preparation to reduce later anxiety is the key.

Q: Are there options for reducing the stress of taking most meals "out"?
A: If it is practical, you could bring your own food, or at least snacks, with you during the trip and select accommodations that allow you to prepare food. For example, if you want to go to a resort, you could pick one where they provide guests with kitchens, so you won't have to depend on outside food services all the time. That is the reason why many parents of allergic children select vacation sites where there is a kitchenette, and they can do their own shopping and prepare their own meals. They may not prepare every meal, but at least they can make some of the meals for themselves or their children using their own preparation rules instead of depending on a restaurant to provide every single meal.

Q: What advice should be followed in regard to foreign travel?
A: When you're traveling to a location where you're not able to converse in the native language with the people providing your meals, you have an additional obstacle. You have to think in advance about how you are going to ask about food in a restaurant setting if you are not able to communicate easily with the individuals who are preparing the food.

For example, you may avoid many concerns by obtaining foods without sauces or flavoring agents and with very simple "whole" ingredients, and by using fresh whole fruits instead of prepared desserts. Still, without the ability to really communicate about meal ingredients and preparation, there would be some risks. Remember also that product labels may pose problems.

Q: Could you use something written down in the native language?
A: You could try that, but there is always a possibility that you think the person has understood what is written, but that person may not really have understood it at all.

A better idea might be to call ahead to the hotel where you will be staying in order to find out what services they provide, whether anyone on the staff speaks English or a language you're familiar with, and how they would approach your instructions about peanut-free meals. If you start looking into this, you may find that some countries appear to be safer than others, and you may want to select one of those for your vacation.

Q: How many self-injectable devices do you have to bring along?
A: My patients typically will ask, "If I'm taking an overseas flight and I'm going to be in the air for twelve hours, or I am going to be far from medical help, how many epinephrine injectors do I need?" In general, most people who experience an allergic reaction will not require more than one dose, and about 10 to 20 percent may need a second dose. As discussed in chapter 13, most of the time it is suggested that you carry two units. This is based on the supposition that the medication gives you time to seek advanced care in an emergency room. Each dose may last roughly

twenty minutes. However, as we previously discussed, you may use a second dose much sooner than that.

The tricky part of answering the question about how many units to take into remote locations is the presumption that advanced care is not available. If someone is extremely ill and not doing well after two doses of epinephrine, he or she probably needs advanced care that is only available from paramedics and an emergency room. If you wanted to calculate one epinephrine unit for every twenty minutes until health care arrived, you would possibly be carrying many units, and if you were ill enough to need more than two or three injections without more care, that would be a bad, though rare, situation.

So the reasonable answer seems to be to have more than your usual number of units, depending upon your travel plans. This could be more than two or three units. Ultimately, it's going to be incredibly important to eat safely and to know exactly what you will do in the event of a reaction. In other words, you have to decide in advance how you will get medical services activated. If you're in a metropolitan area, it's going to be easier than if you're in a remote area.

Q: Is there anything special that should be brought on trips that isn't covered in a regular emergency plan?
A: The emergency action plan and care plan that most peanut-allergic people should carry with them includes:

• Their own knowledge about avoiding the allergen,

• Written materials about their allergies,

• Medical alert bracelets, and

• Antihistamines and self-injectable epinephrine.

You certainly want to have any other needed medication, including inhaled medicines for asthma, if you have asthma. Make sure the medications have not expired. But if you're going to be in very remote areas and an allergic reaction occurs, there is at least one additional medication you may want to have with you: *an oral (taken by mouth) steroid.*

The action of a steroid is described in chapter 15. Briefly, it may quell some of the later aspects of an allergic reaction. Usually, it is not part of an emergency action plan because it does not take effect right away, may not always be needed, and would be available in an emergency room. In the situation of poor access to health care, if you are not able to get medical attention promptly, the steroid could at least give you an extra level of treatment. This is exactly the sort of issue you should discuss with your doctor in regard to exactly where you're going to be and what medical resources will be available to you in that location.

Q: Do you have any advice regarding air travel?
A: In chapter 21, we discussed some of the issues of peanut allergy and casual contact on the airplane. I will briefly review some of the recommendations that are based upon the studies we conducted:

• Be concerned about the practice of actually cooking/ roasting peanuts on an airplane;

• For a child on the airplane, make sure there are no left-over peanuts on the seats or in the seat back pockets, and clean off the tray tables.

• Prepare in advance for the meal, perhaps by bringing a safe meal from home.

• Consider calling ahead for a flight without peanut snacks.

• Consider flying early, when it is less likely peanut will be served.

You can obtain additional information about staying safe on flights from The Food Allergy & Anaphylaxis Network Web site, which typically has information on particular airlines and how they approach peanut allergies (see resources).

Q: Could an airport security guard stop you from bringing your own food and emergency medications on the airplane?
A: That is a possibility in regard to food if you are taking a large amount, particularly internationally, so you should check with your airline in advance about their regulations. In regard to emergency medications, I've taken many flights, and no one has ever stopped me from coming on board with a self-injectable epinephrine device, which I always carry. However, it may make sense to avoid any possible problems by carrying a letter from your doctor stating that you or your child has an allergy and needs to carry this emergency medication in the event of an allergic reaction. A letter like that would probably prevent any issues if the security personnel ask you why you have the medication. In addition, be sure the prescription label is on the device.

29

Psychological Impact, Improving Your Quality of Life, and Teaching Your Children to Manage Peanut Allergy

Q: How do all the considerations about approaching life safely impact an allergic person's quality of life?
A: In my view, living with a peanut allergy is similar to walking through a minefield. Basically, at every meal, the peanut that you are trying so hard to avoid could potentially be in your food and cause a life-threatening reaction. And for many people, living in this minefield can really affect every other aspect of life. The impact is no surprise.

In conjunction with The Food Allergy & Anaphylaxis Network, we have undertaken several studies regarding the impact of food allergy on quality of life, in particular the impact on parents and families of having a food-allergic child. In these studies, we see an impact on people's daily routines. That impact is similar in degree to families who have children with disabilities, such as seizures or chronic arthritis. Specific areas impacted include the very areas discussed in this book, such as school activities, family activities, dining, and shopping. There are also anxieties concerning health and safety.

So the goal is to have as normal a life as possible in the context of having a peanut allergy.

Q: How can people with peanut allergies improve their lives?
A: Hopefully, reading a book like this is one way of trying to do what you can to approach peanut allergy in a reasonable way. In other words, learn all you can about your condition, find out what precautions you need to take, and be vigilant in always doing what is necessary to protect your health and safety. In this way, you can attain a level of control that may reduce anxiety.

Basically, that means you want to do the best you can to minimize risks and maximize your day-to-day activities in terms of enjoying them and living a "normal" life.

For example, I would never tell someone with a peanut allergy not to go to school, not to take a vacation, not to go to their friend's house, or not to have a celebratory dinner. Instead, the idea is to go ahead and do all these things with preparation in mind, reducing your risks as best and as reasonably as you possibly can.

Specific tips to make things easier or to reduce anxiety would vary by your own needs, resources, and abilities. Some of the suggestions include:

- Stay organized. Try to follow a routine that you are comfortable with, and go with previous successes. Use advance preparation to reduce later anxieties (for example, call ahead to restaurants, meet early with schools and camps).

- Spread the responsibilities—one person cannot do everything. Get friends, family, and your spouse involved. Teach your peanut-allergic child to take on age-appropriate responsibilities.

• Don't forget to find time for yourself and your own needs.

• Talk to others living with peanut allergy. You are not alone! And you may learn from their successes, mistakes, and experiences.

If allergic people find they are putting themselves into a bubble where they are afraid to participate in life's activities, that is all the more reason to discuss the problem with their doctors to determine the best approach for them to maximize their ability to get out and do whatever they're supposed to do or whatever they want to do.

Q: Is it easy or even possible to live a normal life with a peanut allergy?
A: Individuals with peanut allergies should be able to achieve all of the same things in life that anyone else does without the peanut allergy preventing them from doing anything—except eating peanut. In my practice, I see some families who are managing extremely well and other families where essentially all the issues are the same, but the impact is enormous. If you feel that you're not able to achieve what you want to, or you are not able to participate in activities when you want to, these situations really have to be addressed. If you are feeling very anxious and worried to a degree that it is affecting your day-to-day activities, that should also be addressed.

Sometimes simply talking over concerns with your doctor, or a friend, or possibly a support group, can help to resolve a concern. Sometimes people with allergies or their families need a professional to help them through these kinds of problems. Fear can become overwhelming, and if that has happened, you should not only discuss it with your primary care doctor and your allergist, but take time to seek additional help from counselors, psychologists, or psychiatrists.

In extreme cases, allergic people can become afraid to eat or afraid to participate in activities. Some of these fears are founded but overgeneralized. And some of these fears may be overcome with simple measures to reduce risks in a reasonable way. With the help of health care professionals, many fearful people can overcome their problems and not have allergies ruin their lives.

Q: Can a peanut allergy actually cause psychological trauma?
A: Having a life-threatening allergy will almost inevitably have a psychological impact. For some people, it motivates them to keep up their guard to insure their own safety but does not prevent them from doing what they wish to do. Unfortunately, for some people it means living in constant fear, with a tangible impact on daily activities. Some fear and anxiety is from the daily focus on the safety of meals and snacks, which are going to be eaten three or more times a day. There is also a fear of being accidentally exposed to a food that can cause severe problems. These conditions can result in allergic people and their families living under constant stress, sometimes leading to psychological problems, ranging from mild to severe.

Then there is additional stress for peanut-allergic people who have experienced a reaction to worry, "Will this happen to me again?" Or, "If it does, could it be worse or even fatal?" So these types of constant worries are quite likely to have an impact and can affect how you view yourself and how you live your life.

Q: How does this stress actually affect everyday lives?
A: In some ways, the psychological condition of people with potentially fatal peanut allergies can be compared to those with post-traumatic stress disorder. People who have been at war and have had a very stressful experience find that when they return to their former lives, their day-to-day living is affected. For example, there's the classic example of someone who's been in a war, is back home, hears a loud noise, and immediately ducks under a table. People with this condition have generalized their horrific experience.

The same type of problems come up in peanut allergy, as well. You may have an individual who has had a life-threatening experience because of peanut, something that other people consider to be a harmless food that's supposed to be a source of nutrition and good health. But for allergic people, it can instead essentially be viewed as a poison. And now they've experienced a severe reaction to it. What's going to happen when they see it on a dining room table? Or smell it on someone's breath? They could actually have an adverse response just because they know they're near something that is life-threatening to them.

The example that I give my patients, which was mentioned perviously, is that if I pull out a gun right now and point it at your head, your heart is going to pound and you're going to sweat and feel like something terrible is happening in your body. That is a normal fear response. It's protective. So people who have experienced a horrific reaction to peanut and then smell or see peanut may well have that same kind of reaction. And even though in a sense it's "normal," it's also something that should be discussed and not something that you would want to overtake your day-to-day living.

Q: What are some of the specific psychological problems you see in relation to peanut allergy?
A: Unfortunately, I sometimes see people who are afraid to go out and participate in life. That means they do not want to face school or work or family activities because of their allergy. I see exactly the post-traumatic stress disorder kinds of responses that were mentioned, in that some people have panic attacks because they are so afraid of a possible exposure to peanut. I also see people who are actually afraid to eat and end up with eating disorders, because they are so frightened that they might accidentally eat something they are allergic to.

Q: How much worry is actually warranted by a peanut allergy?
A: I think that there is a healthy amount of concern, in that you don't want to become lackadaisical about your approach to peanut allergy. For many peanut-allergic people, the condition is potentially severe, and even a small amount can result in a reaction. But those exact words are the same ones that could be counterproductive in terms of moving on with life.

I believe there is a balance that has to be struck, which might be a little bit different for each person's unique personality and allergy. In other words, you have to manage to create a safe environment, while, at the same time, not create an overly restrictive one where you can't do what you want to do.

The solution, therefore, is that you should be properly concerned about your allergy, but that concern should not strangle you.

So if you're going to a restaurant without asking questions because you think you will be able to guess whether the food is safe or not, you are certainly not concerned enough. But if you refuse to eat in any restaurant, you are probably too concerned. The idea is to find a balance between these two extremes that will allow you to live a cautious but normal life.

Q: When should peanut-allergic people seek professional psychological help?
A: That answer may vary from person to person. As mentioned before, if the allergy is stopping you from doing usual activities, impacting your health, or you just feel overly stressed or anxious, you may benefit from professional evaluation.

Q: At what age can children benefit from psychological counseling?
A: In short, the answer is essentially any age. Children or adults of any age group may respond differently to a particular problem over time. For example, a major concern regarding teenagers is that they can be unconcerned about their allergies. They may have spent their childhoods having others worry about the allergy for them, and they only worried about it to a small degree. Then during adolescence, the stereotypical adolescent feeling of "I'm inde-

structible," or "I'm immortal," may take over and become very counterproductive in terms of their taking needed precautions to prevent the ingestion of peanut. Some teens may become anxious or depressed because of their allergy and its restrictions.

Young children, like older individuals, also have a variety of emotional responses. I've seen children become incredibly worried or fearful for their lives. They believe that something horrible is going to happen to them, and they become generally fearful, which is not healthy. So children and adults of any age may have problems that will benefit from psychological counseling.

Q: What should parents teach their children about their allergy?
A: You have to teach your children to protect themselves, in an age-appropriate way, in terms of not sharing food and understanding the symptoms of a reaction, to report symptoms to an adult, and to understand the use of emergency medications. And even though the things that parents teach their children will be individualized according to their child's needs and ability to understand, the precise words a family uses when talking about the allergy with their children should be chosen to take into consideration how their child's general personality might be affected by the allergy.

For example, some families may decide to say, "You can't eat peanuts because they will make you very sick." But they may decide not say to the child, "You'll die if you eat peanuts," because that is a very frightening sentence to use with a young child, and the concept is either going to be very scary or not understood. So with younger children, the burden of keeping the child safe is largely on the family, and they need to explain things to their children in a serious but nonthreatening way that the children can understand.

As children become older, it's important to help them make a transition to a deeper understanding of their allergy and to have them assume more responsibility for protecting themselves.

Q: For the younger children, then, the burden is really on the adults?
A: That's right. The ultimate responsibility is on the supervising adult. This would lead to telling a young child, for example, that "Mommy and Daddy are going to help to keep you safe by doing what we can to try to make sure your food does not have peanut in it, because peanut can make you sick." Notice there is not an absolute promise nor a threat of death for this young child.

But even a young child may be given the responsibility of identifying from whom safe food can be taken. Therefore, you can teach your young child that there are only some adults who know what foods are safe. The child cannot be permitted to think that it is all right to trust just *any* adult when it comes to accepting food. So parents must carefully teach their young children that only the specific adults named by the parents can be trusted in regard to receiving safe food.

In this context, saying "Don't take food from strangers" would *not* be a good way to teach this concept. Most young children do not understand the concept of "stranger," but more importantly, there are likely to be adults who are trusted but not trained for allergy. You should therefore *identify specific adults from whom food can be taken safely* and that food cannot be taken from any other adults.

In other words, you could be walking into a bakery, and the person behind the counter offers your child a cookie. Your child has to be taught in an age-appropriate way that the person in the bakery is not an adult that you said is OK. So the child learns not to accept food from adults who are not peanut-allergy aware, no matter what. They may say, "I cannot take that food because I have a peanut allergy, and my mother has to say what is safe for me to eat."

I think a good way of defining this for young children is to say, "Mommy or Daddy will tell you exactly whom it's OK to take food from, because these are people who know about your allergy. You cannot take food from anyone other than the people we tell you are OK." For example, the parents can tell the child, "Aunt Jane understands what's safe for you to eat, so it is safe for you to take food from Aunt Jane." You can even test your child to reinforce the concept for his or her safety. Have a friend offer your child a treat. If your child takes it, calmly review the concept again. If your child does not take it, praise and reward his or her actions. In all of these situations, explanations and responsibilities must be age-appropriate.

Q: Can you explain what you mean by discussing the allergy in an age-appropriate way?
A: It means that the way you explain an allergy to a child will be different for different children, depending upon their development, and this generally changes as the child gets older. So there isn't any single rule about how to do it or what to say.

For the youngest children, you may want to emphasize, in a simple way:

• Never share food, and

• Only eat food from you (the parent) or an adult you have identified as safe to provide food.

As children get older, the idea of not sharing food can be stressed even more, putting greater responsibility on the children to verbalize the issue. Thus, a transition of responsibility slowly occurs, which is a good thing. The transition is important, because as children are on their own more, they will need to make decisions when their parents and people whom they know are not around, and we need them to make the right decisions.

As they get older, I think it's more useful to tell children the details regarding their peanut allergy and to show them how you, as an adult, make their food safe. In other words, teach them how to read a label. You're not going to have your children buy their own food, but you can bring them shopping with you, so they can see how you're reading labels and selecting which foods to buy. You can begin to let them identify the foods that are safe for them, and maybe give them the reward of picking safe ones they especially want. When you order food at a restaurant, you're doing it for your young child, but you may want a transition to having them discuss the fact that they have a peanut allergy with the restaurant staff, so they can get used to doing it, and it won't be a big deal when they're older.

The main theme here is that parents have to help their peanut-allergic children make transitions so that slowly over time, they take on more and more responsibility for protecting their health and avoiding peanut. This sets up good habits for later years.

Q: Are there support groups for people with peanut allergies?
A: Yes, there are support groups for people with peanut and other food allergies, but at this time, there isn't a huge network of them. (See resources for the Asthma and Allergy Foundation of America, which helps people find support groups.) So, if people want to find a support group, they usually talk to their allergists and ask if there are any local groups. There are also several books rich in advice for families living with a child with food allergies (see resources) and The Food Allergy & Anaphylaxis Network has additional resources.

Case History

THOMAS

Twelve-year-old Thomas had lived with peanut allergy for many years and had become successful in avoiding peanut, but was taking avoidance perhaps too far. Thomas's family had come to see me because they felt their son was becoming overly fearful of peanut exposure to the point that he was limiting his activities because of it.

The family also noticed that Thomas had been washing his hands many times throughout the day; he carried moist towelettes around to wipe doorknobs and furniture, and he had stopped participating in wrestling and other contact sports at school, although he had really enjoyed them in the past. His parents were very concerned that even though Thomas had never had a severe reaction to peanut, he was becoming so frightened of contact with peanut that he was withdrawing from all social contact. All their efforts to change his behavior had failed.

I talked with Thomas and discovered that he was very

worried that there could be some trace of peanut in many things around him, and that he thought about this all day long. He thought that if he did not clean the areas where he was sitting or touching things that he could be contaminated with peanut, even though he understood that it was very unlikely and probably not that great a threat.

After a further discussion with the family, I was informed that some of Thomas's relatives have had obsessive thoughts and compulsive and repetitive behaviors, although the behaviors of the relatives didn't have anything to do with peanut. Perhaps Thomas was exhibiting the same type of obsessive-compulsive behavior.

From my discussions with Thomas and his parents, I concluded that Thomas's obsession with being in contact with peanut was not due to a normal concern about his allergy, nor was it a result of having a peanut allergy, but was a manifestation of the obsessive-compulsive disorder that apparently ran in his family. I reviewed the facts of his allergy with Thomas, explaining that it was very unlikely that casual contact with peanut, such as touching it, could induce a reaction. I explained that in some people, fear can become exaggerated to the point that they need some extra professional help. I suggested that Thomas be evaluated by a psychiatrist.

With treatment, including medication, Thomas was soon able to control his compulsive fears and actions and return to the activities that he had previously enjoyed so much.

Part Five

Looking to the Future

In Part Five, we will look at the studies that are being conducted in an effort to improve both testing and treatment for people with peanut allergies.

30

Future Diagnostic Methods

Q: What are some of the limitations of currently available tests for peanut allergy?
A: I find it very unsatisfying to have patients who may be allergic to peanut and to find that the tests we have done may not be conclusive as to whether or not they actually have a peanut allergy. For example, the allergy skin tests or blood tests may be inconclusive. When that happens, we have to do an oral food challenge, which means we have to feed peanut to the person in order to see whether or not he or she gets sick. No physician wants to make anyone sick. So it would be much better if we had tests that were more definitive without having to feed our patients any peanut.

In the past five years, there has been a dramatic improvement in the allergy tests that are available and in the interpretation of those tests and the results of these improvements have been discussed in chapter 11. So it is a lot more likely that today, as opposed to in the past, we can determine whether or not someone has a peanut allergy without the need to feed peanut to that person. On the other hand, it is still difficult to know for certain whether some of these individuals are really allergic or not. And it is also difficult to know, over time or even at the time of initial diagnosis, whether they will ever outgrow their peanut allergy.

Q: What new developments for better testing and diagnosis are on the horizon?
A: Currently, there are a number of research studies of improved blood tests to see if we can learn more about whether or not someone currently has a true peanut allergy and whether they will outgrow it.

These tests are looking at the different parts of the proteins in peanuts that the body recognizes, and they are trying to find out if the parts that the immune system recognizes on the peanut might give a clue about whether a person is currently allergic or not, and whether they may outgrow the allergy or not.

The other area of diagnosis that is very imperfect is prediction of the severity of a peanut allergy. A lot of families will say to me, "My child has never had a severe reaction. Could he possibly have a severe reaction in the future?"

My answer right now is based primarily on epidemiology, meaning other people's experiences. So if people with peanut allergy have underlying asthma, they are intrinsically at increased risk for a severe reaction from peanut. If they have had a severe reaction in the past, they are intrinsically at increased risk for a having a severe reaction again. But that still leaves a lot of people who don't know what might happen to them. And even within those groups

I just described, we still cannot necessarily predict what will happen.

There are studies going on now that are trying to use a variety of blood tests to decipher whether we can determine if people will have severe or mild reactions. And from some of the preliminary studies, it looks as though that may eventually be possible.

31

Cures and Improved Treatments

Q: What does the future hold for the treatment of peanut allergy?
A: I feel very badly that right now all I have to offer is, "Don't eat peanut, and if you do eat it—and accidents are not unlikely—you need to take medicine to prevent a bad outcome."

In other words, merely offering avoidance and then medical treatment to stamp out fires after an accident has happened is not satisfying for me as a physician and certainly not for people with peanut allergy.

Obviously, what we really want to do is cure the allergy.

There are two basic ways that this goal is currently being studied. One is not necessarily a peanut-specific way of curing allergy, but would instead reduce any type of allergic response. A second way of looking at treating peanut allergy is to create something that cures peanut allergy specifically, rather than all allergies. So the two approaches are:

• Finding a way to cure or reduce all allergies, and

• Finding a way to cure or reduce peanut allergies.

Within these two approaches, there are many different ideas that are being studied, including the development of vaccines and even the use of herbal remedies. Researchers around the world are working on these potential treatments, and a number of strategies are being investigated at the Jaffe Food Allergy Institute at Mount Sinai in New York, where I am doing my research.

Q: Can you tell us more about the possibility of developing a vaccine to treat peanut allergy?
A: The term "vaccine" is a familiar one. For example, there are vaccines to prevent measles or chicken pox. These vaccines are given to change the body's immune response to one that is protective against those specific germs.

When we talk about a vaccine for a peanut allergy, it means that we want the immune system to stop behaving in the wrong way to peanuts and behave the way the immune systems of people without peanut allergy behave.

Just to review some of the concepts discussed earlier, a peanut allergy is an adverse immune response. That means that the part of the body that usually fights infections is essentially attacking the protein in peanut. And we don't want the immune system to do that. So the goal is to get the immune system to see peanut without attacking it.

For example, "allergy shots" or "allergy immunotherapy" is a form of vaccine that is typically given today to people with hay fever. These people are allergic to pollen, and the shot is an injection into the arm of the very same pollen to which they are allergic. Usually when you're exposed to a pollen or animal dander or other things that may cause hay fever or asthma, it gets into your eyes, nose, and lungs, not into your arm. We believe the reason that people have an allergic response is that having the allergen present itself to the body in those places—the eyes, nose, skin, or lungs—leads the immune system to create an allergic kind of response. When the immune system sees the pollen appear in the arm, after weeks and months of repeated injections, it treats the pollen proteins in a different way, a way that gradually becomes a "nonallergic" response.

So if we could inject peanut protein into the arm—just like when we inject pollen or animal dander protein—a whole different part of the immune system will be seeing it and will be treating it differently than it would if it were coming into the body in these other ways. By injecting peanut protein into the arm, we would hope to be able to teach the immune system to treat peanut not like an enemy invader but as something nonthreatening.

Q: Have injections with peanut protein been tried?
A: Giving injections of actual peanut was undertaken in a study years ago, and it actually did work. So people with peanut allergy who got allergy shots with peanut were able to ingest more peanut than they were before the vaccinations, while those on placebo (fake) injections were not improved. Unfortunately, there were also a tremendous number of significant side effects from those shots, and people were actually having allergic reactions to the shots themselves. So it was evident that the side effects of giving peanut-allergic people a shot of peanut vaccine were too strong.

Q: Could there be a way to avoid these side effects?
A: The idea that is being researched now is the creation of a vaccine that does not cause an anaphylactic reaction but still teaches the body to stop attacking peanut, like vaccines or allergy shots for pollen do. One of the strategies to do that involves altering the peanut protein by genetic engineering just enough so that when you inject it, the body still sees it pretty much as peanut protein and could learn to accept it. The idea of this strategy is that by changing the protein a little bit and getting rid of the parts that trigger the IgE or allergic reactions, you would be able to give these types of allergy shots without any side effects, that is, without causing an allergic reaction, and yet still teach the body how to accept peanut and not attack it. At this point in time, this treatment has shown some effectiveness in studies of peanut allergy using mice who are made allergic to peanut and then given this type of treatment to undo the allergy.

Researchers are also considering giving the allergy shot itself with chemicals that trigger a nonallergic immune response. This strategy would possibly heighten and improve the effectiveness of a vaccine.

Q: Are vaccines always shots?
A: Vaccines could be given in a variety of ways. There are vaccines available now that are in the form of nose sprays for the flu, ones taken by mouth for polio, and many others that are in the form of injections or "shots." So there may be a number of different ways of giving a peanut allergy vaccine that may not even require the discomfort of a needle. But all of this has a number of years of investigation, so we will have to wait and see what develops.

Q: How would herbal remedies work?
A: Recently, there have been some published studies using ancient Chinese herbal remedies to try to turn off peanut allergy in mice that were made allergic to peanut. And these herbal remedies seem to be quite effective in the mice.

The treatment involves giving the mice a concoction made from a variety of different herbs. The researcher who created this herbal concoction, Dr. Xiu Min Li at the Jaffe Institute in New York, based it upon what she read about ancient Chinese remedies used for treating illnesses that were somewhat like food allergy. And it did turn out that they were helpful in these mice, but whether they would also be helpful in people is not known at this time. And because we don't know exactly how the herbs work, even in the mice, it's hard to predict what they might do in people and whether they would be safe. So, much more study is going to be required.

Q: Are there other ways to "turn off" the allergic response?
A: A way to try to get the body to stop seeing peanut as a harmful invader is to try to elicit a nonallergic immune response to peanut. That means trying to teach the body to stop looking at peanut as an allergic protein and instead look at peanut in the same way it looks at the many other foods we eat. In other words, get the body's immune system to notice the food but not attack it, as described above in regard to vaccines for allergy.

The hygiene hypothesis, discussed earlier in this book, is the idea that our current way of living does not challenge our immune system with enough "good bacteria." This theory has led to strategies to try to get the body to turn more toward a nonallergic kind of reaction by giving it "good bacteria," or chemicals that come from bacteria. One thought is to combine allergy vaccines with these types of bacteria or bacterial products to get a better nonallergic response. Another strategy has been to give young people "good bacteria" or "probiotics."

Q: What are probiotics?
A: Probiotics are the types of bacteria that we might naturally find in the gut that are not harmful and may actually be beneficial to health, but that we are theorizing are presently either missing or in lower concentrations than might be best for our health. Providing this good bacteria as a supplement to the diet is one general approach to allergy (not just peanut allergy alone) that is being researched.

So far, allergy studies using these treatments were associated with reduced allergic skin rashes in young children prone to such rashes. Whether or not these treatments can help food allergies is not yet known. In fact, in one study that included results of allergy tests to foods, there was no reduction on the allergy test results from using these treatments. However, it was a very small study, and much more needs to be done before we can say whether or not this approach might be helpful.

Q: Is there a way to make a nonallergenic peanut?
A: That is an approach that is also being studied. Researchers are currently looking at genetic engineering in order to see if they can create peanuts that are not allergenic. Since we know what the protein structures in peanut are and how our bodies see those structures, it might be possible to

re-create peanuts without the parts of the proteins that the bodies of those with peanut allergy recognize as enemies. Whether this approach will work remains to be seen.

Q: Are there any viable alternative medicine approaches to peanut allergy?
A: There are a variety of techniques used by individuals that fall under the category of "alternative medicine." But these approaches have not yet been studied in any systematic way, so I can't verify the efficacy or safety of these approaches at this time.

The evidence for them is usually given in the context of studies or descriptions of individual people who had problems with peanut and then were able to have fewer problems with peanut after a variety of modalities were used. These modalities include provocation-neutralization therapy and others. However, the American Academy of Allergy, Asthma and Immunology considers these techniques to be unproven and experimental. My additional concern is that they could be dangerous for patients, and I obviously cannot recommend treatments that have not been proven to be safe and effective.

Q: If peanut allergy isn't cured in the near future, what else might become available to help those with this condition?
A: As I have explained, when you become allergic to peanut or anything else, whether it's another food or something in the environment like a dog or a pollen where sudden allergic reactions may occur from exposure, your body makes molecules called IgE antibodies that are able to detect what you're allergic to. These IgE antibodies float in

the bloodstream and also attach themselves to allergy cells, where they act essentially as antennas. Then, when the offending item comes back into the body, they alert the cells to release the chemicals that cause allergic reactions.

A treatment called "anti-IgE" has been developed and is used for treatment of severe allergic asthma. This treatment is an injected medication given every two to four weeks that attaches itself to these IgE antibodies while they are floating around in the bloodstream, inactivating them. By giving this medication over weeks and months, the IgE antibody that is the troublemaker in all these allergic disorders is sponged away—not completely, but mostly—and therefore causes fewer problems.

This treatment has been very helpful for asthma. The question raised is this: Is the removal or reduction of these IgE antibodies also helpful for people with food allergies? Theoretically, the answer should be "yes." But remember that this therapy removes not only the IgE antibodies that see peanut, but also the ones that see any other food or allergen to which you may be allergic.

The first study to address food allergy with this treatment looked at adults with peanut allergy. The researchers had participants ingest peanut to determine how much was tolerated before a reaction. The participants then received either fake shots (placebos), or actual treatment with an anti-IgE antibody at three different doses. Participants did not know which treatment they were on, and treatments were assigned randomly among the participants. After four months of treatment, peanut was fed again to see how much was tolerated before a reaction developed.

It was observed that people did tolerate more peanut on the treatment, and the higher the dose of treatment, the more they could tolerate. At the highest dose, instead of being able to tolerate an average one-half a peanut, they were able to tolerate nine peanuts, or eighteen times the amount as before.

This was a very exciting result, because people who are avoiding peanut would typically not eat a large amount by accident; they would typically ingest only a small amount. So the idea here is that this approach could provide protection from the small exposures that peanut-allergic people might accidentally get when they were otherwise being careful to avoid peanut.

Q: Were there any negative sides to this study?
A: On the downside of the study was the fact that about one in five of the individuals taking the highest dose had no improvement at all. When they were fed peanut before treatment and then again while on treatment, they reacted to the same amount of peanut, and we do not know why.

Now we are undertaking a similar study with a slightly different formulation than the one used in the original study. We hope to be able to find a dose that is more effective and also determine exactly how protected, or not, people will be with this treatment.

Remember that this is a potential treatment for peanut allergy and not a cure, which means you would have to remain on the therapy indefinitely, and it would serve as a window of safety if you accidentally came across some peanut. But it would not mean that your physician could say, "Go ahead and eat peanuts now, you're protected." Instead, it would be a situation where your physician would say, "You're still going to have to avoid peanut, and you're still going to need to hold on to your emergency medications at all times. But now you're going to be more protected." That is assuming, of course, that the next studies reveal that the treatment works.

It's hard to predict how long it will be before results are available, so it could be a number of years. But we're hoping that this approach will provide a strategy to improve safety for people with peanut allergy and perhaps other allergies as well.

You should also note that this treatment is currently available for those who have allergic asthma and qualify for it for their severe asthma. But you have to remember that if you are on the treatment for allergic asthma and you also happen to have peanut allergy, you should not consider yourself protected from peanut allergy at this point in time, because the dose required for peanut allergy may be completely different or it may turn out not to work. And at this point, we don't yet have that information.

Q: How can someone keep updated in advances in peanut allergy research?
A: Books like this one are very useful, but certain aspects of what we have discussed can become outdated, as there are so many ongoing research studies in peanut allergy and food allergy. In particular, new prevention and treatment strategies may emerge. I therefore encourage the reader to check the Web sites for various organizations listed in the resources section in order to get the most up-to-date information in these areas. In addition, the Web site of the research center where I work is: www.mssm.edu/jaffe_food _allergy.

Conclusion

When you first receive a diagnosis of peanut allergy—whether for yourself or your child—it is overwhelming. You ask yourself, "Why me? What does it mean? How can my family and I ever lead a normal life again?" After all, peanuts are everywhere. Everyone loves peanuts. But suddenly, for you or your child, peanuts have become potentially deadly. This leads to anxiety and many questions about how to be safe and still lead a normal life.

Now that you have read this book, we hope you have found the answers to these and most of your other questions and that you have gained knowledge and understanding that will help you and your family successfully cope with peanut allergy.

It isn't unusual for people to respond to peanut allergy emotionally. Many feel frightened or angry, especially in the early stages. So if you have these feelings, rest assured that your responses are both normal and understandable.

But there is absolutely no need for you or your family to continue to worry indefinitely. As we have seen, virtually all peanut-allergic people can lead active and happy lives, especially if they are very careful to always follow the rules. As we have seen in this book, that means you should:

• Be well-informed. Learn everything you can about peanut allergy and stay up to date by talking regularly to your allergist and doing additional reading and research on your own.

• Be certain that all the people who may supply food or care for you or your peanut-allergic child are also very well-informed. They must all know exactly how to provide protection against the accidental ingestion of peanut and exactly what to do if an accidental ingestion and a reaction do occur.

• Follow all the essential precautions we have discussed in this book, and don't ever let your guard down. As you now know, the most serious reactions can occur when peanut-allergic people are careless, even for a moment. Always be vigilant about avoiding peanut and act promptly if an accidental exposure occurs, so you can protect yourself or your child.

When it comes to dealing with peanut allergy, knowledge is power. When you know what to do and also make sure that all the other people involved in caring for you or your child know as well, you can begin to relax and live a normal, productive life.

Keep reminding yourself that people with peanut allergies can do everything that everyone else does— except eat peanut. They can go to school and birthday parties, take vacations, eat in restaurants, and go away to camp or college. They can participate in sports, play in orchestras and rock bands, win scholarships to top universities, and get married and raise children. They just can't eat peanut.

If the stress of constantly trying to avoid peanut ever becomes too difficult for you or your child to handle, remember that you can always get help from your doctor and from counseling and support groups. Never feel embarrassed about any problems your allergy may cause—living with peanut allergy is definitely not easy!

We all hope that at some time in the near future, medical advances will make peanut allergy a thing of the past. Until that happens, please be careful, stay healthy, and get out there and live!

Resources

WEBSITES AND ORGANIZATIONS (NONPROFIT)

The Food Allergy & Anaphylaxis Network
11781 Lee Jackson Hwy., Suite 160
Fairfax, VA 22033-3309
800-929-4040
www.foodallergy.org

With over 27,000 members, FAAN is a major resource for individuals and families with food allergies. The organization has an internationally recognized medical advisory board that oversees its materials. FAAN offers parent educational conferences; educational books and videos for parents, covering essentially every topic for understanding and managing food allergies; comprehensive programs for preschools, schools, and camps; books for children and teens; and much more. FAAN is also active in education, research, and policy regarding food allergy.

Food Allergy Initiative
237 Park Ave., 21st Floor
New York, NY 10017
212-527-5835
www.foodallergyinitiative.org

This organization's mission includes raising funds to support food allergy research efforts, raising public awareness about food allergy, and improving safety for people with food allergies through education and public policy.

The American Academy of Allergy, Asthma and Immunology
www.aaaai.org
and

The American College of Allergy, Asthma and Immunology
www.acaai.org

These professional organizations have public information resources for allergy and food allergy. In addition, they offer search engines to locate board-certified allergists.

Asthma and Allergy Foundation of America
www.aafa.org

This organization offers numerous resources for people with all types of allergic problems, including information on locating a support group.

Medic Alert
www.medicalert.org

This nonprofit organization offers "linking" the medical identification jewelry to further medical information. There are several competing companies that make medical identification jewelry.

FOR-PROFIT RESOURCES

Dey Pharmaceutical Company
www.EpiPen.com

This Web site has helpful information about anaphylaxis, including a video showing how to use the product this company distributes, the EpiPen.

BOOKS

Caring For Your Child with Severe Food Allergies
Lisa Cipriano Collins, M.A., M.F.T.
John Wiley & Sons, Inc., 2000

This book emphasizes issues associated with the emotional aspects of living with a food allergy.

The Parent's Guide to Food Allergies
Marianne S. Barber
Henry Holt and Company, LLC, 2001

Written by the parent of a child with food allergies, with advice from an allergist and a psychologist, this book provides a wealth of practical information on living with and managing food allergies.

Appendix I

Peanut-Allergic Symptoms

1. Skin
   - Hives
   - Itching
   - Redness
   - Blotches
   - Swelling

2. Lungs/Breathing
   - Congested nose
   - Runny nose
   - Tightening in the throat
   - Swelling of the tongue
   - Difficulty getting air in and out of the throat
   - Constriction or tightening of breathing tubes

3. Gut
   - Itchy mouth
   - Stomach pain
   - Nausea
   - Vomiting
   - Diarrhea

4. Heart
   - Circulation problems
     - Heart not pumping properly
     - Drop in blood pressure, leading to
   - Shock, or a state of poor circulation
     - Paleness
     - Dizziness
     - Disorientation
     - Loss of consciousness
     - Weak pulse

- Feeling of impending
  doom prior to symptoms

- Tingling in the mouth
- Metallic taste in the mouth
- Flushing
- Feeling of impending
  doom

5. Other Symptoms
   - Uterine contractions

NOTE: If you or your child experiences any of the above symptoms after eating peanut and you have not been diagnosed with a peanut allergy, it does not necessarily mean that you have one. However, it is important that you consult a medical professional at the earliest possible moment in order to discover the cause of your symptoms. If you have been diagnosed with a peanut allergy, and you have any of these symptoms, you should follow your doctor's instructions, which are usually to use your medications and go immediately to the nearest emergency room for further evaluation and treatment.

Appendix II

The Peanut-Free Diet

Avoid foods that contain peanut or any of these ingredients:

- Artificial nuts
- Beer nuts
- Cold-pressed, expelled, or extruded peanut oil
- Goobers
- Ground nuts
- Mandelonas
- Mixed nuts
- Monkey nuts
- Nutmeat
- Nut pieces
- Peanut
- Peanut butter
- Peanut flour

May indicate the presence of peanut protein:

- African, Asian (especially Chinese, Indian, Indonesian, Japanese, Thai, and Vietnamese), and Mexican dishes
- Baked goods (pastries, cookies, etc.)
- Candy (including chocolate candy)
- Chili
- Egg rolls
- Enchilada sauce
- Flavoring (including natural and artificial)
- Marzipan
- Nougat

Note: Arachis oil is peanut oil.

NOTE: The above list is not comprehensive, and new products and ingredients constantly appear on the shelves. Therefore, it is very important for you to keep current on such new products and ingredients, to check every product you buy very carefully (every time you buy it, since the label may change), and to avoid purchasing food items in the high-risk stores we have identified, since they may be cross-contaminated with peanut.

Adapted from FAAN, © 2005, The Food Allergy & Anaphylaxis Network, www.foodallergy.org.

Appendix III

Food Allergy Action Plan

Student's
Name:_____ D.O.B:_____ Teacher:_____

ALLERGY TO:_____

Asthmatic Yes* ☐ No ☐   *Higher risk for severe reaction

Place
Child's
Picture
Here

◆ STEP 1: TREATMENT ◆

Symptoms:			Give Checked Medication**:		To be determined by physician authorizing treatment
▪	If a food allergen has been ingested, but *no symptoms*:		☐ EpiPen	☐ Antihistamine	
▪	Mouth	Itching, tingling, or swelling of lips, tongue, mouth	☐ EpiPen	☐ Antihistamine	
▪	Skin	Hives, itchy rash, swelling of the face or extremities	☐ EpiPen	☐ Antihistamine	
▪	Gut	Nausea, abdominal cramps, vomiting, diarrhea	☐ EpiPen	☐ Antihistamine	
▪	Throat †	Tightening of throat, hoarseness, hacking cough	☐ EpiPen	☐ Antihistamine	
▪	Lung †	Shortness of breath, repetitive coughing, wheezing	☐ EpiPen	☐ Antihistamine	
▪	Heart †	Thready pulse, low blood pressure, fainting, pale, blueness	☐ EpiPen	☐ Antihistamine	
▪	Other †	_____	☐ EpiPen	☐ Antihistamine	
▪	If reaction is progressing (several of the above areas affected), give		☐ EpiPen	☐ Antihistamine	

The severity of symptoms can quickly change. † Potentially life-threatening.

DOSAGE
Epinephrine: inject intramuscularly (circle one) EpiPen EpiPen Jr. (see reverse side for instructions)

Antihistamine: give_____
medication/dose/route

Other: give_____
medication/dose/route

◆ STEP 2: EMERGENCY CALLS ◆

1. Call 911 (or Rescue Squad: _____). State that an allergic reaction has been treated, and additional epinephrine may be needed)

2. Dr. _____ at _____

3. Emergency contacts:

Name/Relationship   Phone Number(s)

a. _____   1.)_____   2.)_____

b. _____   1.)_____   2.)_____

c. _____   1.)_____   2.)_____

EVEN IF PARENT/GUARDIAN CANNOT BE REACHED, DO NOT HESITATE TO MEDICATE OR TAKE CHILD TO MEDICAL FACILITY!

Parent/Guardian Signature_____   Date_____

Doctor's Signature_____   Date_____
(Required)

EPIPEN® AND EPIPEN® JR. DIRECTIONS

- **Pull off gray activation cap.**

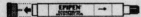

- **Hold black tip near outer thigh (always apply to thigh).**

- **Swing and jab firmly into outer thigh until Auto-Injector mechanism functions. Hold in place and count to 10. Remove the EpiPen® unit and massage the injection area for 10 seconds.**

- **Once EpiPen® is used, call the Rescue Squad. State additional epinephrine may be needed. Take the used unit with you to the Emergency Room. Plan to stay for observation at the Emergency Room for at least 4 hours.**

For children with multiple food allergies, consider providing separate
Action Plans for different foods.

**Medication checklist adapted from the Authorization of Emergency Treatment form developed by the Mount Sinai School of Medicine. Used with permission.*

Appendix IV

School Guidelines for Managing Students with Food Allergies

Food allergies can be life-threatening. The risk of accidental exposure to foods can be reduced in the school setting if schools work with students, parents, and physicians to minimize risks and provide a safe educational environment for food-allergic students.

Family's Responsibility

- Notify the school of the child's allergies.

- Work with the school team to develop a plan that accommodates the child's needs throughout the school, including in the classroom, in the cafeteria, in after-care programs, during school-sponsored activities, and on the school bus, as well as a Food Allergy Action Plan.

- Provide written medical documentation, instructions, and medications as directed by a physician, using the Food Allergy Action Plan as a guide. Include a photo of the child on the written form.

- Provide properly labeled medications and replace medications after use or upon expiration.

- Educate the child in the self-management of his or her food allergy including:

  - Safe and unsafe foods
  - Strategies for avoiding exposure to unsafe foods
  - Symptoms of allergic reactions
  - How and when to tell an adult that he or she may be having an allergy-related problem
  - How to read food labels (age appropriate)

- Review policies/procedures with the school staff, the child's physician, and the child (if age appropriate) after a reaction has occurred.

- Provide emergency contact information.

School's Responsibility

- Be knowledgeable about and follow applicable federal laws including ADA, IDEA, Section 504, FERPA, and any state laws or district policies that apply.

- Review the health records submitted by parents and physicians.

- Include food-allergic students in school activities. Students should not be excluded from school activities solely based on their food allergy.

- Identify a core team of, but not limited to, school nurse, teacher, principal, school food service and nutrition manager/director, and counselor (if available) to work with parents and the student (age appropriate) to establish a prevention plan. Changes to the prevention plan to promote food allergy management should be made with core team participation.

• Assure that all staff who interact with the student on a regular basis understand food allergy, can recognize symptoms, know what to do in an emergency, and work with other school staff to eliminate the use of food allergens in the allergic student's meals, educational tools, arts and crafts projects, or incentives.

• Practice the Food Allergy Action Plan before an allergic reaction occurs to assure the efficiency/effectiveness of the plan.

• Coordinate with the school nurse to be sure medications are appropriately stored, and be sure that an emergency kit is available that contains a physician's standing order for epinephrine. In states where regulations permit, medications are kept in an easily accessible, secure location central to designated school personnel, not in locked cupboards or drawers. Students should be allowed to carry their own epinephrine, if age appropriate, after approval from the student's physician/clinic, parent, and school nurse, and if allowed by state or local regulations.

• Designate school personnel who are properly trained to administer medications in accordance with the state nursing and Good Samaritan laws governing the administration of emergency medications.

• Be prepared to handle a reaction and insure that there is a staff member available who is properly trained to administer medications during the school day, regardless of time or location.

• Review policies/prevention plan with the core team members, parents/guardians, student (age appropriate), and physician after a reaction has occurred.

• Work with the district transportation administrator to assure that school bus–driver training includes symptom awareness and what to do if a reaction occurs.

• Recommend that all buses have communication devices in case of an emergency.

• Enforce a "no eating" policy on school buses with exceptions made only to accommodate special needs under federal or similar laws, or school district policy. Discuss appropriate management of the food allergy with the family.

• Discuss field trips with the family of the food-allergic child to decide appropriate strategies for managing the food allergy.

• Follow federal/state/district laws and regulations regarding sharing medical information about the student.

• Take threats or harassment against an allergic child seriously.

Student's Responsibility

• Should not trade food with others.

• Should not eat anything with unknown ingredients or known to contain any allergen.

• Should be proactive in the care and management of his or her food allergies and reactions based on his or her developmental level.

• Should notify an adult immediately if he or she eats something he or she believes may contain the food to which he or she is allergic.

Developed by The Food Allergy & Anaphylaxis Network in conjunction with the American School Food Service Association, the

National Association of Elementary School Principals, the National Association of School Nurses, and the National School Boards Association. Reprinted with permission from FAAN © 2005, The Food Allergy & Anaphylaxis Network, www.foodallergy.org.

References

Altschul AS, Scherrer DL, Muñoz-Furlong A, Sicherer SH. Manufacturing and labeling issues for commercial products: Relevance to food allergy. *J Allergy Clin Immunol* 2001; 108:468.

American Academy of Pediatrics. Committee on Nutrition. Hypoallergenic infant formulas. *Pediatrics* 2000; 106(2 Pt 1):346–9.

Bernhisel-Broadbent J, Sampson HA. Cross-allergenicity in the legume botanical family in children with food hypersensitivity. *J Allergy Clin Immunol* 1989; 83:435–40.

Bernhisel-Broadbent J, Taylor S, Sampson HA. Cross-allergenicity in the legume botanical family in children with food hypersensitivity. II. Laboratory correlates. *J Allergy Clin Immunol* 1989; 84:701–9.

Beyer K, Ellman-Grunther L, Jarvinen KM, Wood RA, Hourihane J, Sampson HA. Measurement of peptide-specific IgE as an additional tool in identifying patients with clinical reactivity to peanuts. *J Allergy Clin Immunol* 2003; 112(1):202–7.

Bock SA, Atkins FM. The natural history of peanut allergy. *J Allergy Clin Immunol* 1989; 83:900–4.

Burks AW, Bannon GA, Sicherer SH, Sampson HA. Peanut-induced anaphylaxis. *Int Arch Allergy Immunol* 1999; 119:165–72.

Burks AW, King N, Bannon GA. Modification of a major peanut allergen leads to loss of IgE binding. *Int Arch Allergy Immunol* 1999; 118(2–4):313–4.

Burks AW, Shin D, Cockrell G, Stanley JS, Helm RM, Bannon GA. Mapping and mutational analysis of the IgE-binding epitopes on Ara h 1, a legume vicilin protein and a major allergen in peanut hypersensitivity. *Eur J Biochem* 1997; 245(2):334–9.

Busse PJ, Noone SA, Nowak-Wegrzyn AH, Sampson HA, Sicherer SH. Recurrent peanut allergy [Letter]. *N Eng J Med* 2002; 347:1535–6.

Cohen BL, Noone S, Muñoz-Furlong A, Sicherer SH. Development of a questionnaire to measure quality of life in families with a food-allergic child. *J Allergy Clin Immunol* 2004; 114(5):1159–63.

Eigenmann PA, Burks AW, Bannon GA, Sampson HA. Identification of unique peanut and soy allergens in sera adsorbed with cross-reacting antibodies. *J Allergy Clin Immunol* 1996; 98:969–78.

Emmett SE, Angus FJ, Fry JS, Lee PN. Perceived prevalence of peanut allergy in Great Britain and its association with other atopic conditions and with peanut allergy in other household members [published erratum appears in *Allergy* 1999 Aug; 54(8):891]. *Allergy* 1999; 54(4):380–5.

Ewan PW. Clinical study of peanut and nut allergy in 62 consecutive patients: New features and associations. *BMJ* 1996; 312(7038):1074–8.

Fleischer DM, Conover-Walker MK, Christie L, Burks AW, Wood RA. Peanut allergy: Recurrence and its management. *J Allergy Clin Immunol* 2004; 114(5):1195–201.

Fleischer DM, Conover-Walker MK, Christie L, Burks AW, Wood

RA. The natural progression of peanut allergy: Resolution and the possibility of recurrence. *J Allergy Clin Immunol* 2003; 112(1):183–9.

Foucard T, Malmheden YI. A study on severe food reactions in Sweden—is soy protein an underestimated cause of food anaphylaxis? *Allergy* 1999; 54(3):261–5.

Frick OL, Teuber SS, Buchanan BB, Morigasaki S, Umetsu DT. Allergen immunotherapy with heat-killed *Listeria* monocytogenes alleviates peanut and food-induced anaphylaxis in dogs. *Allergy* 2004; DOI111.

Furlong TJ, DeSimone J, Sicherer SH. Peanut and tree nut allergic reactions in restaurants and other food establishments. *J Allergy Clin Immunol* 2001; 108:867–70.

Golding J, Fox D, Lack G. Prevalence and natural history of peanut allergy in children in the UK. *J Allergy and Clin Immunology* 1998; 101:S103.

Grundy J, Matthews S, Bateman B, Dean T, Arshad SH. Rising prevalence of allergy to peanut in children: Data from 2 sequential cohorts. *J Allergy Clin Immunol* 2002; 110(5): 784–9.

Gu X, Simons K, Solver N, Johnston L, Simons F. Epinephrine injection (EpiPen Jr vs EpiPen) in young children at risk for anaphylaxis. *J Allergy and Clin Immunol* 2001; 107: S58.

Hallett R, Haapanen LA, Teuber SS. Food allergies and kissing. *N Engl J Med* 2002; 346(23):1833–4.

Hayami D, Kagan R. The positive predictive value of prick skin tests to peanut in children who have never previously eaten peanuts. *J Allergy Clin Immunol* 2000; 105:S189.

Hefle SL, Lemanske RFJ, Bush RK. Adverse reaction to lupine-fortified pasta. *J Allergy Clin Immunol* 1994; 94(2 Pt 1):167–72.

Hoffman DR, Collins-Williams C. Cold-pressed peanut oils may contain peanut allergen. *J Allergy Clin Immunol* 1994; 93:801–2.

Hourihane JOB, Bedwani SD, Dean TP, Warner JO. Randomized double-blind crossover challenge study of allergenicity of peanut oils in subjects allergic to peanuts. *BMJ* 1997; 314:1084–88.

Hourihane JO, Dean TP, Warner JO. Peanut allergy in relation to heredity, maternal diet, and other atopic diseases: Results of a questionnaire survey, skin prick testing, and food challenges. *BMJ* 1996; 313(7056):518–21.

Hourihane JO, Kilburn SA, Nordlee JA, Hefle SL, Taylor SL, Warner JO. An evaluation of the sensitivity of subjects with peanut allergy to very low doses of peanut protein: A randomized, double-blind, placebo-controlled food challenge study. *J Allergy Clin Immunol* 1997; 100(5):596–600.

Hourihane JO, Roberts SA, Warner JO. Resolution of peanut allergy: Case-control study [see comments]. *Br Med J* 1998; 316(7140):1271–5.

Isolauri E, Rautava S, Kalliomaki M, Kirjavainen P, Salminen S. Role of probiotics in food hypersensitivity. *Curr Opin Allergy Clin Immunol.* 2002 Jun 2;(3)263–71.

Jones RT, Stark D, Sussman G, Yunginger JW. Recovery of peanut allergens from ventilation filters of commercial airliners (abstract). *J Allergy Clin Immunol* 1996; 97:423.

Joshi P, Mofidi S, Sicherer SH. Interpretation of commercial food ingredient labels by parents of food allergic children. *J Allergy Clin Immunol* 2002; 109:1019–21.

Kalliomaki M, Salimen S, Poussa T., Arvilommi H, Isolauri E. Probiotics and prevention of atopic disease: 4-year follow-up of a randomized placebo-controlled trial. *Lancet.* 2003 May 31; 361(9372):1869–71.

Keating MU, Jones RT, Worley NJ, Shively CA, Yunginger JW.

Immunoassay of peanut allergens in food-processing materials and finished foods. *J Allergy Clin Immunol* 1990; 86:41–4.

Kelso JM. Resolution of peanut allergy. *J Allergy Clin Immunol* 2000; 106(4):777.

Kelso JM, Connaughton C, Helm RM, Burks W. Psychosomatic peanut allergy. *J Allergy Clin Immunol* 2003; 111(3): 650–1.

Kemp SF, Lockey RF. Peanut anaphylaxis from food cross-contamination [letter]. *JAMA* 1996; 275(21):1636–7.

Lack G, Fox D, Northstone K, Golding J. Factors associated with the development of peanut allergy in childhood. *N Engl J Med* 2003; 348(11):977–85.

Lee SY, Huang CK, Zhang TF, Schofield BH, Burks AW, Bannon GA, et al. Oral administration of IL-12 suppresses anaphylactic reactions in a murine model of peanut hypersensitivity. *Clin Immunol* 2001; 101(2):220–8.

Legendre C, Caillat-Zucman S, Samuel D, Morelon S, Bismuth H, Bach JF, et al. Transfer of symptomatic peanut allergy to the recipient of a combined liver-and-kidney transplant. *N Engl J Med* 1997; 337(12):822–4.

Leung DYM, Sampson HA, Yunginger JW, Burks W, Schneider LC, Shanahan W. Effect of anti-IgE therapy (TNX-901) in patients with severe peanut allergy. *N Engl J Med* 2003; 348:986–93.

Leung DY, Shanahan WR, Jr., Li XM, Sampson HA. New approaches for the treatment of anaphylaxis. *Novartis Found Symp* 2004; 257:248–60.

Lever LR. Peanut and nut allergy: Creams and ointments containing peanut oil may lead to sensitisation. *BMJ* 1996; 313(7052):299.

Li XM, Sampson HA. Novel approaches to immunotherapy for food allergy. *Clin Allergy Immunol* 2004; 18:663–79.

Li XM, Srivastava K, Grishin A, Huang CK, Schofield B, Burks W et al. Persistent protective effect of heat-killed *Escherichia coli* producing "engineered" recombinant peanut proteins in a murine model of peanut allergy. *J Allergy Clin Immunol* 2003; 112(1):159–67.

Li XM, Srivastava K, Huleatt JW, Bottomly K, Burks AW, Sampson HA. Engineered recombinant peanut protein and heat-killed *Listeria* monocytogenes coadministration protects against peanut-induced anaphylaxis in a murine model. *J Immunol* 2003; 170(6):3289–95.

Li XM, Zhang TF, Huang CK, Srivastava K, Teper AA, Zhang L, et al. Food Allergy Herbal Formula-1 (FAHF-1) blocks peanut-induced anaphylaxis in a murine model. *J Allergy Clin Immunol* 2001; 108(4):639–46.

Macdougall CF, Cant AJ, Colver AF. How dangerous is food allergy in childhood? The incidence of severe and fatal allergic reactions across the UK and Ireland. *Arch Dis Child* 2002; 86(4):236–9.

Maleki SJ, Chung SY, Champagne ET, Raufman JP. The effects of roasting on the allergenic properties of peanut proteins. *J Allergy Clin Immunol* 2000; 106(4):763–8.

Matheu V, de Barrio M, Sierra Z, Gracia-Bara MT, Tornero P, Baeza ML. Lupine-induced anaphylaxis. *Ann Allergy Asthma Immunol* 1999; 83(5):406–8.

Mittag D, Akeerdaas J, Ballmer-Weber B, et al. Ara h 8 a Bet v 1 homologous allergen from peanut is a major allergen in patients with combined birch pollen and peanut allergy. *J Allergy Clin Immunol*. 2004; 114:1410–17.

Moneret-Vautrin DA, Guerin L, Kanny G, Flabbee J, Fremont S, Morisset M. Cross-allergenicity of peanut and lupine: The risk of lupine allergy in patients allergic to peanuts. *J Allergy Clin Immunol* 1999; 104(4 Pt 1):883–8.

Moneret-Vautrin DA, Kanny G, Morisset M, Flabbee J, Guenard

L, Beaudouin E et al. Food anaphylaxis in schools: Evaluation of the management plan and the efficiency of the emergency kit. *Allergy* 2001; 56(11):1071–6.

Moneret-Vautrin DA, Rance F, Kanny G, Olsewski A, Gueant JL, Dutau G et al. Food allergy to peanuts in France—evaluation of 142 observations. *Clin Exp Allergy* 1998; 28(9):1113–19.

Morisset M, Moneret-Vautrin DA, Kanny G, Guenard L, Beaudouin E, Flabbee J et al. Thresholds of clinical reactivity to milk, egg, peanut and sesame in immunoglobulin E-dependent allergies: Evaluation by double-blind or single-blind placebo-controlled oral challenges. *Clin Exp Allergy* 2003; 33:1046–51.

Muraro A, Dreborg S, Halken S, Host A, Niggemann B, Aalberse R et al. Dietary prevention of allergic diseases in infants and small children: Part III. Critical review of published peer-reviewed observational and interventional studies and final recommendations. *Pediatr Allergy Immunol* 2004; 15(4): 291–307.

Nowak-Wegrzyn A, Conover-Walker MK, Wood RA. Food-allergic reactions in schools and preschools. *Arch Pediatr Adolesc Med* 2001; 155(7):790–5.

Oppenheimer JJ, Nelson HS, Bock SA, Christensen F, Leung DYM. Treatment of peanut allergy with rush immunotherapy. *J Allergy Clin Immunol* 1992; 90:256–62.

Pascual CY, Fernandez-Crespo J, Sanchez-Pastor S, Padial MA, Diaz-Pena JM, Martin-Munoz F et al. Allergy to lentils in Mediterranean pediatric patients. *J Allergy Clin Immunol* 1999; 103(1 Pt 1):154–8.

Perry TT, Conover-Walker MK, Pomes A, Chapman MD, Wood RA. Distribution of peanut allergen in the environment. *J Allergy Clin Immunol* 2004; 113(5):973–6.

Perry TT, Matsui EC, Conover-Walker MK, Wood RA. The relationship of allergen-specific IgE levels and oral food challenge outcome. *J Allergy Clin Immunol* 2004; 114(1):144–9.

Pons L, Ponnappan U, Hall RA, Simpson P, Cockrell G, West CM et al. Soy immunotherapy for peanut-allergic mice: Modulation of the peanut-allergic response. *J Allergy Clin Immunol* 2004; 114(4):915–21.

Pucar F, Kagan R, Lim H, Clarke AE. Peanut challenge: A retrospective study of 140 patients. *Clin Exp Allergy* 2001; 31(1):40–6.

Pumphrey RS. Fatal anaphylaxis in the UK, 1992–2001. *Novartis Found Symp* 2004; 257:116–28.

Pumphrey RS. Fatal posture in anaphylactic shock. *J Allergy Clin Immunol* 2003; 112(2):451–2.

Pumphrey RS, Nicholls JM. Epinephrine-resistant food anaphylaxis. *Lancet* 2000; 355(9209):1099.

Rance F, Abbal M, Lauwers-Cances V. Improved screening for peanut allergy by the combined use of skin prick tests and specific IgE assays. *J Allergy Clin Immunol* 2002; 109(6):1027–33.

Rhim GS, McMorris MS. School readiness for children with food allergies. *Ann Allergy Asthma Immunol* 2001; 86(2):172–6.

Sampson HA. Clinical practice: Peanut allergy. *N Engl J Med* 2002; 346(17):1294–9.

Sampson HA. Managing peanut allergy. *BMJ* 1996; 312(7038):1050–1.

Sampson HA. Peanut anaphylaxis. *J Allergy Clin Immunol* 1990; 86:1–3.

Sampson HA. Utility of food-specific IgE concentrations in predicting symptomatic food allergy. J Allergy Clin Immunol 2001; 107(5):891–6.

Sampson HA, Mendelson LM, Rosen JP. Fatal and near-fatal anaphylactic reactions to food in children and adolescents. N Engl J Med 1992; 327:380–4.

Shreffler WG, Beyer K, Chu TH, Burks AW, Sampson HA. Microarray immunoassay: Association of clinical history, in vitro IgE function, and heterogeneity of allergenic peanut epitopes. *J Allergy Clin Immunol* 2004; 113(4):776–82.

Sicherer SH. Beyond oral food challenges: Improved modalities to diagnose food hypersensitivity disorders. *Curr Opinion Allergy Clin Immunol* 2003; 3:185–8.

Sicherer SH. Clinical implications of cross-reacting food proteins. *J Allergy Clin Immunol* 2001; 108:881–90.

Sicherer SH. Diagnosis and management of childhood food allergy. *Current Problems in Pediatrics* 2001; 31:35–57.

Sicherer SH. Food allergy. *Lancet* 2002; 360:701–10.

Sicherer SH. Food challenges: When and how to perform oral food challenges. *Pediatr Allergy Immunol* 1999; 10:226–34.

Sicherer SH. Manifestations of food allergy: Diagnosis and treatment. *Am Family Physician* 1998;59:415–24.

Sicherer SH. New insights on the natural history of peanut allergy [editorial]. *Ann Allergy Asthma Immunol* 2000; 85:435–7.

Sicherer SH. Peanut Allergy: A clinical update. *Ann Allergy Asthma Immunol* 2002; 88:350–61.

Sicherer SH. Self-injectable epinephrine: One size does not fit all [Editorial]. *Ann Allergy Asthma Immunol* 2001; 86:597–8.

Sicherer SH. The impact of maternal diet during breast-feeding on the prevention of food allergy. *Curr Opinion Allergy Clin Immunol* 2002; 2:207–10.

Sicherer SH, Burks AW, Sampson HA. Clinical features of acute allergic reactions to peanut and tree nuts in children [full article, electronic access]. *Pediatrics* 1998; 102:E6.

Sicherer SH, Burks AW, Sampson HA. Peanut and soy allergy: A diagnostic and therapeutic dilemma. *Allergy* 2000; 55:515–21.

Sicherer SH, Forman JA, Noone SA. Use assessment of self-administered epinephrine among food allergic children and pediatricians. *Pediatrics* 2000; 105:359–62.

Sicherer SH, Furlong TJ, DeSimone J, Sampson HA. Self-reported peanut allergic reactions on commercial airlines. *J Allergy Clin Immunol* 1999; 104:186–9.

Sicherer SH, Furlong TJ, DeSimone J, Sampson SH. Peanut allergic reactions in schools. *J Pediatr* 2001; 138:56–65.

Sicherer SH, Furlong T, Maes HH, Desnick RJ, Sampson HA, Gelb BD. Genetics of peanut allergy: A twin study. *J Allergy Clin Immunol* 2000; 106:53–6.

Sicherer SH, Furlong TJ, Muñoz-Furlong A, Burks AW, Sampson HA. A Voluntary registry for peanut and tree nut allergy: Characteristics of the first 5,149 registrants. *J Allergy Clin Immunol* 2001; 108:138–42.

Sicherer SH, Morrow EH, Sampson HA. Dose-response in double-blind, placebo-controlled food challenges in children with atopic dermatitis. *J Allergy Clin Immunol* 2000; 105:582–6.

Sicherer SH, Muñoz-Furlong A, Burks AW, Sampson HA. Prevalence of peanut and tree nut allergy in the US determined by a random digit dial telephone survey. *J Allergy Clin Immunol* 1999; 103:559–62.

Sicherer SH, Muñoz-Furlong A, Sampson HA. Prevalence of peanut and tree nut allergy in the US determined by a random digit dial telephone survey: A five year follow-up Study. *J Allergy Clin Immunol* 2003; 112:1203–7.

Sicherer SH, Noone SA, Muñoz-Furlong A. The impact of childhood food allergy on quality of life. *Ann Allergy Asthma Immunol* 2001; 87:461–64.

Sicherer SH, Sampson HA. Food allergy emergencies. *Office and Emergency Pediatrics* 1999;12:140–7.

Sicherer SH, Sampson HA. Peanut and tree nut allergy. *Curr Opinion Ped* 2000; 12:567–73.

Sicherer SH, Teuber SS. Academy Practice Paper: Current approach to the diagnosis and management of adverse reactions to foods. *J Allergy Clin Immunol* 2004; 114(5):1146–50.

Simons FE. Advances in H1-antihistamines. *N Engl J Med* 2004; 351(21):2203–17.

Simons FE. First-aid treatment of anaphylaxis to food: Focus on epinephrine. *J Allergy Clin Immunol* 2004; 113(5):837–44.

Simons FE, Chan ES, Gu X, Simons KJ. Epinephrine for the out-of-hospital (first-aid) treatment of anaphylaxis in infants: Is the ampule/syringe/needle method practical? *J Allergy Clin Immunol* 2001; 108(6): 1040–4.

Simons FE, Gu X, Silver NA, Simons KJ. EpiPen Jr versus EpiPen in young children weighing 15 to 30 kg at risk for anaphylaxis. *J Allergy Clin Immunol* 2002; 109(1):171–5.

Simons FE, Gu X, Simons KJ. Epinephrine absorption in adults: Intramuscular versus subcutaneous injection. *J Allergy Clin Immunol* 2001; 108(5):871–3.

Simonte SJ, Ma S, Mofidi S, Sicherer SH. Relevance of casual contact to peanut butter in peanut-allergic children. *J Allergy Clin Immunol* 2003; 112:180–3.

Skolnick HS, Conover-Walker MK, Barnes-Koerner C, Sampson HA, Burks AW, Wood RA. The natural history of peanut allergy. *J Allergy Clin Immunol* 2001; 107: 367–74.

Spergel JM, Beausoleil JL, Pawlowski NA. Resolution of childhood peanut allergy. *Ann Allergy Asthma Immunol* 2000; 85(6 Pt 1):473–6.

Sporik R, Hill D. Allergy to peanut, nuts, and sesame seed in Australian children [letter]. *BMJ* 1996; 313(7070):1477–8.

Sporik R, Hill DJ, Hosking CS. Specificity of allergen skin testing in predicting positive open food challenges to milk, egg and peanut in children. *Clin Exp Allergy* 2000; 30(11):1541–6.

Tariq SM, Stevens M, Matthews S, Ridout S, Twiselton R, Hide DW. Cohort study of peanut and tree nut sensitisation by age of 4 years. *BMJ* 1996; 313(7056):514–7.

Taylor SL, Busse WW, Sachs MI, Parker JL, Yunginger JW. Peanut oil is not allergenic to peanut-sensitive individuals. *J Allergy Clin Immunol* 1981; 68:372–5.

Taylor SL, Hefle SL, Bindslev-Jensen C, Atkins FM, Andre C, Bruijnzeel-Koomen C et al. A consensus protocol for the determination of the threshold doses for allergenic foods: How much is too much? *Clin Exp Allergy* 2004; 34(5): 689–95.

Taylor SL, Hefle SL, Bindslev-Jensen C, Bock SA, Burks AW, Jr., Christie L et al. Factors affecting the determination of threshold doses for allergenic foods: How much is too much? *J Allergy Clin Immunol* 2002; 109(1):24–30.

TenBrook JA, Wolf MP, Hoffman SN, et al. Should beta-blockers be given to patients with heart disease and peanut-induced anaphylaxis? A decision analysis. *J Allergy Clin Immunol* 2004; 113:977–82.

Teuber SS, Brown RL, Haapanen LA. Allergenicity of gourmet nut oils processed by different methods. *J Allergy Clin Immunol* 1997; 99(4):502–7.

Teuber SS, Del Val G, Morigasaki S, Jung HR, Eisele PH, Frick OL et al. The atopic dog as a model of peanut and tree nut food allergy. *J Allergy Clin Immunol* 2002; 110(6):921–7.

Vadas P, Perelman B. Activated charcoal forms non-IgE binding complexes with peanut proteins. *J Allergy Clin Immunol* 2003; 112(1):175–9.

Vadas P, Wai Y, Burks W, Perelman B. Detection of peanut allergens in breast milk of lactating women. *JAMA* 2001; 285(13):1746–8.

Vander Leek TKJ, Liu AH, Bock SA. The natural history of peanut allergy in young children and its association with peanut-specific IgE [abstract]. *J Allergy Clin Immunol* 2000; 105:S187.

Vierk K, Falci K, Wolyniak C, Klontz KC. Recalls of foods containing undeclared allergens reported to the US Food and Drug Administration, fiscal year 1999. *J Allergy Clin Immunol* 2002; 109(6):1022–6.

Warner JO. Peanut allergy: A major public health issue. *Pediatr Allergy Immunol* 1999; 10(1):14–20.

Wensing M, Knulst AC, Piersma S, O'Kane F, Knol EF, Koppelman SJ. Patients with anaphylaxis to pea can have peanut allergy caused by cross-reactive IgE to vicilin (Ara h 1). *J Allergy Clin Immun* 2003; 111:420–4.

Wensing M, Penninks AH, Hefle SL, Koppelman SJ, Bruijnzeel-Koomen CA, Knulst AC. The distribution of individual threshold doses eliciting allergic reactions in a population with peanut allergy. *J Allergy Clin Immunol* 2002; 110(6):915–20.

Yunginger JW, Ahlstedt S, Eggleston PA, Homburger HA, Nelson HS, Ownby DR, Platts-Mills TA, Sampson HA, Sicherer SH, Weinstein AM, Williams PB, Wood RA, Zeiger RS Quantitative IgE antibody assays in allergic diseases. *J Allergy Clin Immunol* 2000;105:1077–84.

Zeiger RS. Food allergen avoidance in the prevention of food allergy in infants and children. *Pediatrics* 2003; 111(6 Pt 3):1662–71.

Zimmerman B, Urch B. Peanut allergy: Children who lose the positive skin test response. *J Allergy Clin Immunol* 2001; 107(3):558–9.

About the Authors

Scott H. Sicherer, M.D., is associate professor of pediatrics at the Mount Sinai School of Medicine and a researcher in the Jaffe Food Allergy Institute at Mount Sinai. Dr. Sicherer received his medical degree with honors from the Johns Hopkins University School of Medicine, and his pediatric training, including a chief residency, at Mount Sinai in New York City. He completed a fellowship in allergy and immunology at Johns Hopkins and then returned as faculty to Mount Sinai. Dr. Sicherer is board-certified in pediatrics and in allergy and immunology and specializes in food allergies. He cares for children with food allergies at the Jaffe Food Allergy Institute at the Mount Sinai School of Medicine in New York City. His research interests, funded by the National Institutes of Health, the USDA, the Food Allergy Initiative, and The Food Allergy & Anaphylaxis Network, include allergic diseases caused by specific foods, such as peanuts, tree nuts, and milk, the natural history of food allergy, atopic dermatitis, gastrointestinal manifestations of food allergies, psychosocial issues associated with food allergies, and the genetics of food allergy. Dr. Sicherer has published over ninety articles on food allergy, including original research, scientific reviews, and book chapters. He is a medical advisor to The Food Allergy & Anaphylaxis Network, The Food Allergy Initiative, and others. He is past chair of the Adverse Reactions to Foods Committee of the American Academy of Allergy, Asthma and Immunology. He is on the editorial board of the *Journal of Allergy and Clinical Immunology*. Dr. Sicherer lives with his wife and their five children in New Jersey.

Terry Malloy is a freelance writer specializing in health and medical issues, whose previous books include *Liposuction* (Berkley, 2004) and *Botox* (Berkley, 2002), both written with Ron M. Shelton, M.D.; *Creatine and Other Natural Muscle Boosters* (Dell, 1999), written with Robert Monaco, M.D.; and *Viagra: The Wonder Drug for Peak Performance* (Dell, 1999), written with E. Douglas Whitehead, M.D. Also a screenwriter, Terry Malloy lives in suburban New York.